The Dental Teacher

R. M. Baiju • Sabu Thomas
Editors

The Dental Teacher

A Reference Guide to Instructional Strategies and Evaluation Principles

Springer

Editors
R. M. Baiju
Periodontology, Professor and PhD Guide
Government Dental College
Kottayam, Kerala, India

Kerala University of Health Sciences
Thrissur, Kerala, India

Sabu Thomas
International and Interuniversity Centre
for Nanosciences
Mahatma Gandhi University
Kottayam, Kerala, India

ISBN 978-3-032-07550-5 ISBN 978-3-032-07551-2 (eBook)
https://doi.org/10.1007/978-3-032-07551-2

This Springer imprint is published by the registered company Springer Nature Switzerland AG
The registered company address is: Gewerbestrasse 11, 6330 Cham, Switzerland

To all passionate dental teachers

Foreword by K. Nandakumar

It is with great pride and deep satisfaction that I write the foreword to this insightful and much-needed book titled "*The Dental Teacher*" on teaching-learning methodology and its application for dental professional teachers. The book is coedited by my student R. M. Baiju, who himself is an acclaimed dental teacher and Prof Sabu Thomas—a world-renowned scientist and educationist. This work represents not only an exceptional academic contribution to dental education but also a heartfelt commitment to improving how we train the next generation of dental health professionals.

Throughout my career as a dental educator and educational administrator, I have witnessed first-hand the challenges that even an experienced teacher face in the dynamic world of professional dental teaching. Dentistry is a fast-changing world. With technology integration, there is a growing need for student-centred learning. The focus has shifted from teaching, which was teacher centred, to learning, which puts the student at the centre. With improved and equitable access to the internet and technology becoming more affordable to the common man, every discipline is witnessing an information revolution. Teacher is not the sole information provider and learning no longer is restricted to the class rooms or clinics. The emphasis now is on self-directed and self-paced learning. This change has made it imperative for dental teachers to refine the teaching methods and upskill periodically to keep pace with the changing student's needs. In this context, *The Dental Teacher* is an admirable step forward. The editors and contributors have thoughtfully reviewed every evidence-based methodology and analysed the practical application of the same.

The sound balance between theory and practice sets this book apart. It is not just about mere discussion on pedagogical concepts; rather it offers insightful action plans set in a realistic dental school environment. The editor's approach is marked by clarity, simplicity, and depth. The book aspires to enhance both teaching and learning experiences for teachers at all levels of the career ladder.

I commend Prof R. M. Baiju and Prof Sabu Thomas for undertaking this endeavour with utmost sincerity, academic rigour, and a futuristic perspective. I am confident that this book will, for sure, serve as a valuable reference source for dental educators, educational administrators, curriculum planners, and students alike.

I congratulate the authors and sincerely wish the readers a pleasant and worthwhile reading experience through the pages ahead.

K. Nandakumar

Azeezia College of Dental Sciences
Kollam, Kerala, India
Department of Periodontology
Government Dental College
Thiruvananthapuram, Kerala, India

Foreword by R. Sajith Kumar

The field of education is drastically changing for the better in all disciplines all over the world. Competency-Based Dynamic Curriculum (CBDE) has been introduced by regulatory bodies in many countries. Competency is the expression of fitness for practice, which is expected to escalate to competence in community environment. Competency-Based Dental Education aims at bringing better dental graduates contributing to better oral health in the country.

Several countries including the USA, Canada, Australia, and the UK have formulated a holistic competency framework for a dental graduate. With globalisation of the economy and countries witnessing increasing migration of skilled professionals including doctors and dentists, there is an urgent need for dental schools and universities to ensure that their curriculum is in accordance with the global competency framework. Capacity building of the dental teachers and periodic upskilling should be an important agenda. Any new change always attracts resistance, in spite of the benefits associated. Significant number of teachers in medical and dental streams have not undergone any specific training in teaching learning methodology in general and handling the CBDE curriculum in particular. Besides the changing scenarios incorporating self-learning, online learning, artificial intelligence, etc. are making the learning environment entirely different from the student days of our teachers. The onslaught of cognitive material available now at fingertips for students and teachers alike makes classroom learning less important. Along with that, there are incidents being reported where the soft skills of professionals are being challenged by the changing society as well. Thus, Change has become the keyword in all dimensions of human life not sparing the dental college campuses as well.

This changing scenario demands change in attitudes, behaviour, skills, and practice of our teachers. This is being addressed in a miniscule level by certain teacher training programmes. However, well-formulated reference material or faculty guide is yet to see light. This attempt by the authors of this book is well appreciated. Readers will definitely find each sentence in this book enlightening and stimulating. This endeavour is sure to make the mindset of teachers brighten up with new ideas being triggered, which will benefit the upcoming young students and graduates to be more skilled, responsive, and empathetic professionals who will become good team leaders and lifelong learners. All this will ultimately translate to welfare of the common man, to which category, each one of us belong.

Best wishes to the authors, personnel behind this great activity, faculty, and readers.

R. Sajith Kumar

Acknowledgements

With deep gratitude, we acknowledge the tremendous encouragement and support received from all those who were involved in making this book. The book was conceptualised to provide a simple and engaging read to a professional dental teacher irrespective of his/her stature or work experience. We are blessed to rope in the best minds to contribute the chapters according to their expertise. All the contributors are vastly experienced dental educators with decades of experience in dental teaching, and some are senior academic administrators involved in curriculum planning and evaluation. We express our heartfelt gratitude to all contributors for their dedication and the tremendous effort they have put in the making of this book.

We express our sincere thanks to our colleagues in the Department of Periodontics and International and Inter University Centre for Nano Sciences, Mahatma Gandhi University, Kottayam. The research scholars and postgraduate students of both centres have put in their valuable time and effort to the successful completion of this book. Their cooperation and unconditional support will be remembered for a long time.

Words are not enough to thank our colleagues and friends who have helped us with the peer review of the submitted manuscripts. We wish to acknowledge Dr Santhosh Kumar S, Dr Tony Kurien, Dr Rekha P R, Dr Mohammed Shereef, and Dr Neethu P Reghu of Department of Peridontics, Government Dental College, Kottayam. Thanks are also due to Dr Hanna and Dr Joshy of the Mahatma Gandhi University, Kottayam.

Special thanks to Dr R Sajith Kumar and Dr K Nandakumar for willingly agreeing to pen the foreword. Dr K Nandakumar is a role model dental teacher who have taught thousands of dental graduates and hundreds of specialists for more than 40 years. Dr Sajith Kumar is a pioneer in medical education technology in the country. He played a pivotal role in designing and implementing the competency-based dynamic medical curriculum for National Medical Commission in 2018. Both the doyens have mentored hundreds of medical and dental teachers including several contributors of this book.

We would like to specially mention Dr Kannan V, Principal, Government Dental College, Kottayam, for his constant encouragement.

We thank our publishers for their professionalism, perseverance, and tolerance that helped us to complete this project.

Last but not the least we thank our lovely families for their sacrifice, understanding, love, and care without which this work wouldn't have been possible.

R. M. Baiju
Sabu Thomas

Contents

Contributors

Taniya Rose Abraham School of Energy Materials, Mahatma Gandhi University, Kottayam, Kerala, India

Adejumoke A. Adeyemi School of Dentistry, Institute of Life Course and Medical Sciences, University of Liverpool, Liverpool, UK

R. M. Baiju Government Dental College, Kottayam, Kerala, India
Kerala University of Health Sciences, Thrissur, Kerala, India

K. Chandrasekharan Nair AECS Maaruthi College of Dental Sciences, Bangalore, India
Sree Sankara Dental College, Thiruvavanthapuram, India

A. Devadathan Pushpagiri Institute of Dental Sciences, Thiruvalla, Kerala, India
Faculty of Dentistry, Kerala University of Health Sciences, Thrissur, Kerala, India

K. Harikumar Department of Periodontics, Government Dental College Kozhikode, Kozhikode, Kerala, India

K. P. Jayachandran School of Nanoscience and Nanotechnology, Mahatma Gandhi University, Kottayam, Kerala, India
School of Pure and Applied Physics, Mahatma Gandhi University, Kottayam, Kerala, India

N. D. Jayakumar Saveetha University, Chennai, India

Saju Joseph School of Nanoscience and Nanotechnology, Mahatma Gandhi University, Kottayam, Kerala, India

Vinod Krishnan Department of Orthodontics, Sri Sankara Dental College, Thiruvananthapuram, Kerala, India
Kerala University of Health Sciences, Thrissur, Kerala, India

Vivek Narayan Public Health Dentistry, Government Dental College, Kottayam, Kerala, India
Kerala University of Health Sciences, Thrissur, Kerala, India

Claire Newey School of Dentistry, Institute of Life Course and Medical Sciences, University of Liverpool, Liverpool, UK

Elbe Peter Government Dental College, Thrissur, Kerala, India
Kerala University of Health Sciences, Thrissur, Kerala, India

P. R. Rekha Department of Periodontics, Government Dental College, Kottayam, Kerala, India

R. Sajith Kumar Department of Infectious Diseases, Convener NMC Nodal Centre for Faculty Development, Government Medical College, Kottayam, Kerala, India
Academic Staff College, Kerala University of Health Sciences, Thrissur, Kerala, India

Anil Sukumaran Oral Health Institute, Periodontics, Hamad Medical Corporation, DOHA, Qatar
College of Dental Medicine, Qatar University, DOHA, Qatar

Nidhitha Suresh Saveetha University, Chennai, India

Biju Thomas Department of Periodomtology, AB Shetty Memorial Institute of Dental Sciences, Nitte University, Mangalore, India

Sabu Thomas International and Interuniversity Centre for Nanosciences, Mahatma Gandhi University, Kottayam, Kerala, India

Teaching and Learning in Dentistry: The Current Paradigm

1

R. M. Baiju

1.1 Introduction

The twenty-first century has witnessed one of the greatest pandemics of all times—the COVID-19 pandemic. Human life and everything related to living have changed after the commencement of the pandemic. The unprecedented pandemic had a huge impact on all walks of human life including healthcare administration, education, employment and economics. We all have witnessed the paradigm change the pandemic brought about in the global education sector in general and the medical and dental education in particular. The prevailing concept of public health is founded on the biopsychosocial model. Hence, health is dependent upon multiple factors. Changes in human behaviour influence general health of people. The rapid pace of industrial development, advancement in technology, population growth, transcontinental migration and the resultant economic and environmental impact have led to the emergence of new diseases and conditions. This will have a profound impact on the healthcare needs of the society. The expectations and needs of the society regarding healthcare eventually dictate revisions to the existing medical education programmes.

Traditionally there have been two models of dental education—the odontology and stomatology models. The odontology model perceives dentistry as an autonomous discipline with an independent curriculum from medicine, although there are many common shared domains which are inseparable. This approach is prevalent in Northern and Western Europe, America, Australia, Japan and India. However, the stomatology model, prevalent primarily in some parts of Europe and in China, recognises dentistry as a specialty of medicine. The professional programme for dental undergraduate courses is a well-structured one in world's most leading universities. The dental undergraduate professional programme is broadly divided as preclinical,

R. M. Baiju (✉)
Government Dental College, Kottayam, Kerala, India

Kerala University of Health Sciences, Thrissur, Kerala, India

R. M. Baiju, S. Thomas (eds.), *The Dental Teacher*,
https://doi.org/10.1007/978-3-032-07551-2_1

paraclinical and clinical segments in most countries. The first half of the course is dedicated to teaching medical basic sciences relevant to the practice of dentistry. Dental surgery involves utilisation and manipulation of a lot of laboratory materials and biomaterials. The first 2 years are spent on learning about the dental material science. There is no uniformity in the curricula taught in different parts of the world and hence there is no universal criterion for establishing the competence of a dental graduate. However, there are core attributes leading to clinical competence identified by international professional bodies of dentistry. Better informed patients, improved access to healthcare and the Internet revolution providing health-related information at their fingertips have transformed healthcare practice and delivery.

1.2 What Has Changed in Dental Education?

Since the last decade of the previous century, the concept of consumerism has influenced the doctor-patient relationships. Patients are now better informed about their rights and privileges. There has been a marked improvement in health awareness and good lifestyle practices. With the advancement in communication technology and the emergence of high-speed Internet, working hours have increased exponentially, eroding personal time. People tend to avoid healthcare visits due to pressures to strike a work-life balance. Facilities for online consultations and telemedicine have fuelled this change.

Similar to William Osler's famous quote 'medicine is learnt at the bedside', it can be rightly said that dentistry is learnt at the chairside. Dental students learn from direct patient contact and the shared lived experience of patients. Clinical training of a dental student involves multiple levels of patient engagement in pursuit of imparting clinical procedural skills and communication skills. Patients, thus, are an indispensable component in the clinical training triad, the other two being students and teachers.

The treatment clinics attached to dental schools offer a unique situation in that they provide dental care by unlicensed dental students under the supervision of qualified teaching clinicians [1]. Although the treatment cost is low, the process is time-consuming as each step requires supervisory checks by the licensed teaching clinician. The patients who visit the teaching hospitals are contributing to the sustenance of the dental profession by selflessly serving as teaching aids. There has been a tremendous increase in the number of medical and dental schools in most countries and there is a proportional increase in access to healthcare even in the remotest parts of the world, although there is still a long way to go in terms of fulfilment of the broad and somewhat elusive concept of *health for all.* Consequently, there is a considerable decrease in patient availability in tertiary care teaching hospitals for clinical teaching, putting medical and dental teachers as well as their students at a disadvantage. To address this, some dental schools have come up with dedicated priority clinics to provide personalised, prompt service to patients. But this facility is literally detached from the teaching environment, as dental teaching does not happen here.

The issue of generation gap is real. The difference between two generations stems from difference in opinion and attitudes towards social, cultural, religious, political, moral and ethical values and beliefs. The students in dental schools are different from those who were there when the present-day dental teachers were studying. The virtual learning environment is increasing its stake in dental education in current times. Modern-day students consider themselves partners in education and masters of their own learning. With the access to information at their fingertips, self-directed learning and self-paced learning are the new standards.

The role of the teacher has changed. The traditional role of a teacher as an information provider has become obsolete. The modern-day dental teacher rather recognises the information overload as a problem. He or she has to identify, evaluate and organise recommendable pieces of learning material for the benefit of the students who, on the other hand, are perplexed with the sea of information available with the press of a button. The classic article by Ronald Harden and Crosby, pioneers in medical education technology, has illustrated 12 different roles of a teacher [2]. The teacher has become primarily a learning facilitator and coach, although there are multiple other roles to be performed. With increasing access to information, breathtaking progress in information communication and technology, the needs, aspirations and expectations of the dental student of the new millennium.

It is different and demanding. The curriculum requires major revisions and the teaching-learning environment must equip itself to cater quality education relevant to modern times. Dentistry has witnessed tremendous progress in the twenty-first century, driven by advancements in the understanding of the pathologic mechanisms of important dental health conditions. Advancements in therapeutic strategies, including promising strides in regenerative medicine, aesthetic dentistry and CAD/CAM design, have positioned dentistry strategically in the wellness industry as well. To keep pace with the growth of the dental industry, teaching and learning in dental schools should have to evolve in order to prepare the next generation competent dentists.

1.3 The Issue of Globalisation of Dental Education

Post COVID, the higher education sector has opened and an aspiring dental student can learn dentistry in any part of the world. Due to uneven distribution of dentists in different parts of the globe and rising unemployment or under employment, there is a rise in the transmigration of dental graduates across continents. It goes without saying that, in order to comply with the local legal and ethical regulations, the dental graduate has to match the standards prescribed by the migrating country. In other words, dental schools should strive to provide a uniform dental curriculum across various universities that is globally relevant. This may be achieved with international collaborations, opening multiple campuses in various countries and student exchange programmes.

In lieu of globalisation, there is a huge difference in the economic landscape of the world. Formerly economic giants have become less powerful and new countries including China and India have become more prosperous [3]. This throws open new possibilities in consumer demand in such countries. The oral healthcare industry has not reached its full potential within the new economic powers and the consumer demand appears to be unmet to a larger extent. The dental education sector in such countries requires major revisions to meet the improved societal demand in the aftermath of globalisation and economic reforms. Constant liaison with all stakeholders is warranted to create a dynamic educational framework that is capable of adapting to changing needs.

1.4 Quality Assurance and Accreditation in Dental Education

In pursuit of providing value-based and quality education, higher education centres and universities are relying on internal as well as external quality assurance initiatives. There are agencies that provide training and assessment of systems and processes in ensuring standards and metrics in dental professional training. Accreditation agencies agree upon an internationally accepted benchmarking in performance auditing and quality assurance. It assesses the performance of teachers and students, periodic evaluation of teaching and learning activities, infrastructure, extracurricular collaborations, industry and community engagements and innovations with respect to the discipline of interest. It helps students, educational administrators and the public alike in knowing the position and progress of a particular programme in a learning institute in comparison to local as well as global rankings. This has instilled a healthy competition among top institutes to strive to achieve excellence in their performance. This augurs well for the aspiring students and parents. There is another side to this as most teachers consider accreditation as an additional job for them, contributing to their exhaustion and burnout.

Periodic performance assessment of dental educators is required to fine-tune their workmanship and professionalism. Student feedback is an integral aspect of most quality assurance initiatives in dental education. Safe disposal of biomedical waste without affecting climate change is a big task. The next generation of dental health professionals has to be trained to resort to healthier, safer and environmentally friendly practices in biomedical waste disposal.

1.5 Student Burn Out and Academic Stress

A conducive learning environment that safeguards students' self-esteem and confidence is paramount in an educational process of building clinical competence [4]. Such positive behaviour is crucial in empowering students to interact actively with peers and engage with faculty for an improved learning experience. Academic stress is rampant in many higher education centres and dental schools are no exception. Studies show that not only busy practitioners experience burnout; even a first-year dental student can fall prey for this menace. Up to 43% of medical students have reported to suffer from considerable academic stress [5]. Dental schools follow a residency training programme wherein students have to stay within the campus away from the comfort and support of their homes. This, along with the packed schedule of lectures, demonstrations, practical and skill training and patient care, contribute immensely to burnout. Alarmingly, suicidal ideation is also reported to be around 11% among medical students, especially those who suffer from considerable academic stress [6]. Students experiencing coping issues with the demanding academic responsibilities may resort to substance abuse, which will have a strong negative impact on their performance scores. Students' well-being is paramount for any institution and more so for dental schools. Systems have to be in place to recognise this issue and remedial measures have to be instituted. Mentorship and psychological counselling are a newer addition to the existing roles of the dental teacher. Expert medical intervention has to be resorted to when needed. Modern-day dental schools consider this as an important issue that is critical to students' welfare inside the campus and have systems to address this. Right from needs assessment to programme evaluation, in all steps of curriculum development, measures are adopted to minimise academic stress and to provide an enjoyable learning experience to students.

Students and their families also must be aware of the student burnout. Pre-admission education and counselling programmes targeted at potential candidates can be beneficial. Those who seek admission to dental graduate course should have the right aptitude and attitude to meet the challenges of the dental syllabus, which calls for physical exertion, artistry and an enterprising attitude to successfully crack and win the course.

1.6 Educational Research

Medical education technology is an established and rapidly advancing science with quality content being published from sincere and sound workplace-based research. In comparison to niche journals on medical education, there are only very few journals of international repute on dental education. Two important journals focusing on dental education are the *Journal of Dental Education* and the *European Journal of Dental Education*. A few general dentistry journals like the *British Dental Journal* have sections dedicated to dental education. A bibliometric analysis of research papers based on dental education reports that research papers on dental education are listed among the top 100 most cited articles [7]. To improve the efficiency and effectiveness of educational strategies and to devise new strategies, dental schools and universities have to foster more research initiatives in educational methodology. In order to enhance research capacity, collaborations may be established with other related educational research streams such as medicine. Dental teaching faculties who pursue educational research have to be encouraged by the provision of time and money. A research-enabling environment has to be created within dental schools to encourage educational research activities.

1.7 What Needs to Change?

1.7.1 Inconsistency Among Teachers in Teaching and Assessment

The students identified four major areas of concern about their dental education: (1) lack of efficiency and resultant unproductive time in the clinical environment; (2) instructional strategies of some faculty who emphasised teaching and testing for memorisation; (3) interactions with a segment of the faculty who exhibited poor teaching methods and/or poor attitudes; and (4) a widespread perception of inconsistency among instructors during assessment of student performance (comprising feedback, ratings, and grades).

1.7.2 Periodic Curriculum Revision

Many universities function under an established hierarchy in an overly rigid framework. The coarse curriculum is established based on a systematic process beginning with a needs assessment. Curriculum revision is based on societal demand. In reality, being a labourious and labour-intensive process, curriculum revision does not happen as intended. This leads to redundant content being taught time and again in spite of resentment from both teachers who deliver the syllabus and students who receive it. In a competency-based educational system, dynamism has to be established in curriculum implementation and delivery.

1.7.3 Induction Training for Faculty and Regular Faculty Training

In dental schools, we teach students who are over 18 years, hence they are adults. In 1984, Knowles described how adult learners differ from children. According to him, pedagogical skills are not enough to teach and engage adult learners. The adult learner brings with him life experiences that have a profound impact on how and what they learn. Knowles has described the process of adult learning as *androgogy*. Adult learners are self-directed and self-motivated, often aware of how and what he/she learns. It is significant to understand about learner types and their behaviour. All those who teach, including those who teach pre-primary classes, must mandatorily undergo formal training and be certified before employment. Any professional, whether skilled or not, with the right aptitude or not, can teach in a dental school, according to prevailing norms. Faculty development is critical to curricular development. Accreditation agencies mandate dental teachers to get trained once in every 2 or 3 years to ensure work-based standards. Induction training and periodic skill enhancement courses for faculty may be instituted to improve the general teaching and learning standards in dental schools. Medical education technology has now become a full-blown science, and it highlights the importance of training medical and dental teachers and future teachers.

Among the different roles of a teacher, assessment is an integral aspect. Standardised, non-biased assessment of students' learning is essential in ensuring quality assurance in the process as well as product. The examination process should have the virtues of reliability, validity and objectivity. Teachers should be willing for self-development in order to meet the demands of the next generation of dental students.

Most dental schools follow a traditional compartmentalised teaching strategy where in students are posted in various clinical departments in a pre-determined order. Students attend clinics in one specialty for a few weeks continuously and then they move to the next in the process. This fragmented teaching style may deprive them of the opportunity to understand the generalist concept of treatment. A comprehensive assessment of the patient's dental health issues may not be addressed and taught in this approach. Rather, training to formulate a patient-centred care plan in a comprehensive clinical set-up may go a long way in building the required clinical competencies in the student.

1.7.4 Teacher-Student Ratio

The teacher-student ratio is skewed with more students and fewer teachers per student. For proper implementation of teaching strategies and ensuring fair and formal student assessment, a sufficient number of teachers are necessary. The student-teacher contact and the quality time spent by the teacher with students are paramount in the making of professional attributes in a dental student. Dental schools have to recruit a greater number of qualified personnel in their professional training faculty. Regulatory bodies should insist on stringent guidelines to effect this change.

Introducing better integration and interdisciplinary approaches is suggested to improve the teaching-learning activities in professional dental schools. In an outcome-based approach, the end point is the making of a competent professional who is ready for practice. Both horizontal and vertical integration in the teaching of different subjects have to be strategised and implemented for better learning in a more realistic clinical environment.

A study from the University of Texas, United States, conducted among dental students, reports that students consider the initial pre-clinical period of study in the curriculum as a hurdle before their clinical training [8]. In comparison to medical students, dental students will be providing certain irreversible clinical procedures in a conscious patient under the monitoring and supervision of their clinical teachers. In this context, early exposure of dental students to the clinical environment may be more motivating to them and may sow the seeds within them of self-direction and ownership in their learning.

1.7.5 Online Education

One of the takeaways of the recent pandemic is the introduction of an online mode of teaching and learning. In spite of its inherent drawbacks, the online mode has added a new dimension to education. Universities have identified those sections of the syllabus that can be taught online. It may vary from discipline to discipline, but it is a possibility even in medicine and dentistry where, a lot of psychomotor and affective skills training is imparted. Curriculum planners now increasingly recognise this possibility and map courses or portions of them that can be delivered online or through hybrid mode. The online learning mode helps learners to overcome the constraints of time and space. Certain courses can be learned in a self-paced manner, as it suits all kinds of learners, including slow learners and advanced learners. There is a huge potential for online learning management systems in the future in imparting value-based education for a larger audience who are sitting remotely from the learning centre.

References

1. Nalliah RP. Could dental school teaching clinics provide better care than regular private practices? J Investig Clin Dent. 2019;10:e12329.
2. Harden RM, Crosby JR. AMEE education guide no 20: the good teacher is more than a lecturer—the twelve roles of the teacher. Med Teach. 2000;22(4):334–47.
3. Sharma S, Vijayaraghavan V, Tandon P, Kumar DRV, Sharma H, Rao Y. Dental education: current scenario and future trends. J Contemp Dent Pract. 2012;13(1):107–10.
4. Blegur J, Tlonaen Z, Lumba A, Leko J. The importance of self-esteem to students learning responsibilities and group learning commitment of physical education students. JETL. 2021;6:53.
5. Saten SA, Holt DB, Jemp JD, Hemphill RR. Burnout in medical students: examining the prevalence and associated factors. South Med J. 2010;103(8):758–63.
6. Dyrbye LN, Thomas MR, Huntington JL, Lawson KL, Novotny PJ, Sloan JA, Shanafelt TD. Personal life events and medical student burnout: a multicenter study. Acad Med. 2006;81(4):374–84. https://doi.org/10.1097/00001888-200604000-00010. PMID: 16565189
7. Kandaswamy E. Areas of interest in dental education: a bibliometric analysis of the last decade. Cureus. 2024;16(5):e59589. https://doi.org/10.7759/cureus.59589. PMID: 38826921; PMCID: PMC11144435
8. Henzi D, Davis E, Jasinevicius R, Hendricson W. In the students' own words: what are the strengths and weaknesses of the dental school curriculum? J Dent Educ. 2007;71(5):632–45. PMID: 17493972

Educational Goals and Objectives in Dental Education

2

Anil Sukumaran

2.1 Introduction

The landscape of dental education in India has evolved substantially since the establishment of the first dental college in Calcutta in 1920. Today, with over 300 dental colleges producing approximately 25,000 graduates annually, India has one of the largest dental education systems globally. However, this quantitative growth necessitates a parallel qualitative advancement through well-defined educational goals and objectives [1]. This chapter explores the theoretical foundations, practical applications and cultural contexts of academic goals and objectives tailored explicitly for the Bachelor of Dental Surgery (BDS) curriculum in Indian universities. Educational goals and objectives serve as the compass guiding dental education in India. They provide a framework for defining what students should learn, how they should know and how their learning will be assessed. In essence, they are the roadmap to creating competent, ethical and compassionate dental professionals who can meet the oral healthcare needs of the diverse Indian population [2]. Dentistry stands at the intersection of science, art and patient care. Its practitioners are entrusted with preserving and restoring oral health and improving their patients' overall quality of life. In this intricate and evolving domain, the foundation of dental education is pivotal—built upon carefully crafted educational goals and objectives that serve as the guiding light for educators and learners.

2.1.1 Role of Goals and Objectives in Dental Education

The importance of well-defined educational goals and objectives cannot be overstated. They provide clarity and focus for curriculum design, teaching methodologies and assessment strategies, helping dental educators concentrate on what truly

A. Sukumaran (✉)
Oral Health Institute, Periodontics, Hamad Medical Corporation, DOHA, Qatar

College of Dental Medicine, Qatar University, DOHA, Qatar

R. M. Baiju, S. Thomas (eds.), *The Dental Teacher*,
https://doi.org/10.1007/978-3-032-07551-2_2

matters in preparing future dentists. They establish accountability and transparency—making it possible to evaluate whether educational outcomes are being met by all stakeholders—students, faculty, institutions and regulatory bodies such as the Dental Council of India. Furthermore, they facilitate continuous improvement as they evolve with advancements in dental science, technology and the changing oral healthcare needs of Indian society [3].

2.1.2 Unique Challenges and Opportunities in Indian Dental Education

2.1.2.1 Challenges

The Indian dental education system navigates a complex landscape shaped by the country's unique socioeconomic and demographic characteristics. With a population exceeding 1.4 billion people dental educators face the monumental task of addressing extraordinarily diverse oral health needs, spanning from remote rural villages to sophisticated urban centres. This diversity creates a challenging educational environment where future dentists must be prepared to treat patients across vastly different socioeconomic backgrounds with varying access to preventive care. Infrastructure and resource disparities among dental institutions further complicate the educational landscape. Whilst premier dental colleges boast state-of-the-art facilities and experienced faculty, many institutions struggle with inadequate clinical equipment, outdated learning resources and insufficient student-patient exposure. These disparities create an uneven quality of dental graduates across the country [4].

The rapid pace of technological advancement in dentistry presents another significant challenge. Due to financial constraints, many dental colleges face difficulties integrating cutting-edge technologies—such as digital dentistry, CAD/CAM systems and advanced imaging techniques—into their curricula. This technological gap can leave graduates underprepared for modern dental practice environments. Further complicating matters is the ongoing 'brain drain' phenomenon, where talented dental educators and researchers are drawn to international opportunities offering better compensation and research facilities [5]. This exodus of expertise creates faculty shortages in Indian dental institutions—potentially compromising educational quality and research output.

2.1.2.2 Opportunities

The Indian dental education sector is poised for significant growth, driven by several encouraging trends. The general population's rising awareness of oral health has created unprecedented demand for quality dental services across urban and rural areas. This expanding market offers dental graduates diverse career opportunities—from establishing private practices to joining corporate dental chains or pursuing specialised roles in emerging fields such as cosmetic and digital dentistry. Government support has become increasingly robust, with initiatives like the National Oral Health Programme and the integration of dental health into broader healthcare policies. These programmes improve public oral health and create structured frameworks for dental education enhancement, research funding and rural outreach programmes that benefit educational institutions.

Technology adoption is revolutionising dental education in India. Digital learning platforms, virtual patient simulations and AI-assisted diagnostic training make quality dental education more accessible and standardised nationwide. Institutions that embrace these innovations can overcome traditional infrastructure limitations and provide students with cutting-edge learning experiences despite physical resource constraints [6]. Perhaps most exciting is India's extraordinary potential as a dental research hub. The country's vast population presents diverse clinical scenarios, genetic variations and unique oral health challenges—creating an unparalleled environment for groundbreaking research. Dental institutions that capitalise on this advantage can contribute significantly to global oral health knowledge whilst elevating India's position in international dental academia.

2.2 Theoretical Frameworks for Educational Goals and Objectives

Educational goals represent broad, long-term educational outcomes that guide the overall direction of a curriculum or programme. They articulate what students should achieve by the completion of their dental education. They often align with the institution's core values and the dental profession's broader expectations. For example, a common educational goal in dentistry is to prepare graduates who can provide high-quality, patient-centred care whilst addressing the oral health needs of diverse populations [7]. Objectives, in contrast, are specific, measurable statements that describe knowledge, skills or attitudes students should demonstrate after completing a learning activity or course. They break down the larger aspirations into actionable steps, providing a clear framework for curriculum design, teaching and assessment. For instance, an educational objective might be to ensure that students can demonstrate proficiency in diagnosing and treating common dental conditions by the end of their clinical training. In the Indian dental education context, goals and objectives must align with the guidelines established by the Dental Council of India (DCI) whilst addressing the unique healthcare needs of India's diverse population.

2.2.1 Understanding the Hierarchy: Goals vs. Objectives

Understanding the difference between educational goals and objectives is essential for designing and implementing effective dental education programmes. Goals are overarching visions that reflect the long-term aspirations of a programme. They are broad, abstract and often qualitative, focusing on the 'why' and 'what' of education. For example, a goal might be to produce graduates who are leaders in the field of dentistry capable of advancing the profession through innovation and research. In contrast, objectives are specific, measurable and actionable steps that outline the 'how' of achieving these goals (Table 2.1). They are concrete and often quantifiable, providing clear criteria for assessing student performance. For instance, an objective might be to ensure that students can perform a root canal procedure with 90% accuracy by the end of their training. The relationship between goals and objectives is hierarchical [8]. Goals provide the overarching vision whilst objectives break down that vision into manageable tasks. This hierarchical structure ensures that the curriculum is aligned with the programme's mission and that students are systematically prepared to meet the profession's expectations.

2.2.2 *Bloom's Taxonomy* in Dental Education

Bloom's Taxonomy provides a hierarchical framework for classifying educational objectives into three primary domains: cognitive, affective and psychomotor (Fig. 2.1). This framework is particularly valuable in dental education, where practitioners must develop comprehensive knowledge, professional attitudes and precise clinical skills [9].

2.2.2.1 Cognitive Domain (Knowledge)

The cognitive domain encompasses intellectual skills, progressing from basic recall to complex critical thinking and creation. **Remember** represents the foundation of cognitive skills—involving recalling facts and basic concepts. In dental education, this manifests as recalling the anatomical structures of the oral cavity. **Understanding** builds on this foundation, requiring students to explain ideas or concepts. Dental students demonstrate understanding when they can explain the pathophysiology of periodontal disease. **Apply** involves using the information in new situations. This is evident when students select appropriate dental materials for specific clinical scenarios. **Analysis** requires drawing connections among ideas. In dental contexts, this might involve differentiating between various types of malocclusion. **Evaluation** entails justifying a stand or decision. Dental students engage in evaluation when critically assessing treatment outcomes. **Create** the highest cognitive level, involves producing new or original work. This is demonstrated when students develop comprehensive treatment plans for complex cases.

Table 2.1 Educational hierarchy: goals and objectives in dental curriculum design

Characteristics	Educational goals	Educational objectives
Scope	Broad, overarching	Specific, narrow focus
Timeframe	Long-term	Short to medium-term
Specificity	General statements	Precise, measurable statements
Focus	The 'why' and 'what'	The 'how'
Measurability	Often qualitative	Quantifiable
Example	'Produce graduates who can address the oral health needs of diverse populations'	'By the end of the periodontics course, students will perform scaling and root planing with 90% accuracy'

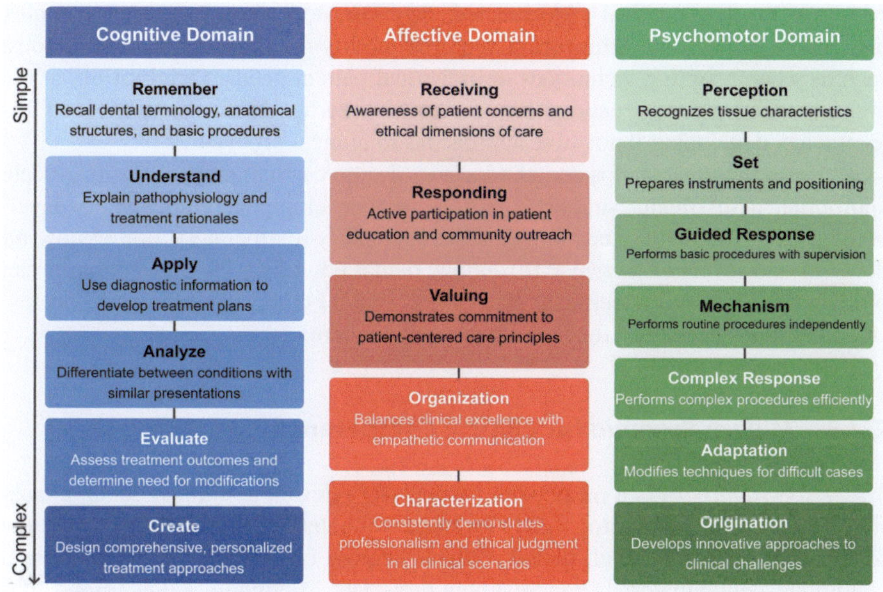

Fig. 2.1 *Bloom's Taxonomy* applied to dental education. This illustration comprehensively applies *Bloom's Taxonomy* across all three learning domains within dental education

2.2.2.2 Affective Domain (Attitudes)

The affective domain addresses emotional aspects of learning, including feelings, values, appreciation, enthusiasm, motivations and attitudes. **Receiving** forms the base level, involving awareness and willingness to hear. Dental students demonstrate this when being attentive to infection control protocols. **Responding** moves beyond awareness to active participation. This is demonstrated when students actively participate in community dental health programmes.

Valuing represents the acceptance of a value. In dental education, this emerges when students demonstrate commitment to ethical practice. **Organisation** involves organising values into priorities. Students reach this level when integrating professional values with personal beliefs. **Characterisation** represents the highest level where values are internalised. This is evident when students embody patient-centred care in all professional interactions.

2.2.2.3 Psychomotor Domain (Skills)

The psychomotor domain is crucial in dentistry, encompassing physical movement, coordination and motor skills. **Perception** begins with sensory awareness, such as recognising changes in tissue texture. **Set** involves a readiness to act, demonstrated when students correctly position instruments for a procedure. **Guided response** represents the early stage of learning a skill, which is evident when students follow a procedure under direct supervision. **Mechanism** signifies the intermediate skill development stage when students confidently perform routine procedures. **Complex**

response involves skillful performance, demonstrated when executing complex procedures efficiently. **Adaptation** requires modifying skills for new situations, such as when adapting techniques to individual patient needs. **Origination**, at the highest level, involves creating new movement patterns. Dental students reach this level when developing innovative approaches to clinical procedures.

Bloom's Taxonomy helps dental educators design curriculum progression, create appropriate assessments, support comprehensive development, guide faculty development and facilitate student self-assessment. By deliberately addressing all domains and levels of *Bloom's Taxonomy*, dental education [10] programmes can produce graduates with technical proficiency, critical thinking abilities and professional attitudes necessary for high-quality patient care.

2.2.3 *Miller's Pyramid* for Clinical Competence

Miller's Pyramid offers a framework particularly relevant to clinical dental education by establishing four progressive levels of competence development [11]. At the foundational 'Knows' level, dental students acquire factual knowledge about oral conditions, dental materials and treatment protocols. Moving to 'Knows How', students learn to apply this knowledge by understanding diagnostic reasoning and treatment planning for various dental scenarios. The 'Shows How' level involves demonstrating clinical skills in preclinical laboratories and simulated environments, where students practise procedures on mannequins before patient contact. Finally, at the 'Does' level, students perform independently on actual patients under supervision, integrating knowledge, skills and professional attitudes [12]. This framework is especially valuable in the Indian context, where dental students must transition from theoretical understanding to clinical competence whilst adapting to limited resources and addressing the diverse oral health needs of varied patient populations with different socioeconomic backgrounds and cultural beliefs about dental care (Fig. 2.2).

2.2.4 SMART Objectives in Dental Education

Educational objectives in dental education must adhere to the SMART (Specific—Measurable—Achievable—Relevant—Timebound) criteria to effectively guide teaching and learning processes, ensuring clarity, accountability and meaningful outcomes for educators and students. The **specificity criterion** requires objectives to identify the exact knowledge, skill or attitude students should demonstrate, avoiding vague language and delineating the scope and boundaries of expected performance. This precision eliminates ambiguity and enables students to focus their learning efforts appropriately. **Measurability** transforms objectives from aspirational statements into practical assessment tools by incorporating quantifiable criteria or observable behaviours that provide concrete evidence of achievement. These measurement parameters might include accuracy percentages, error rates,

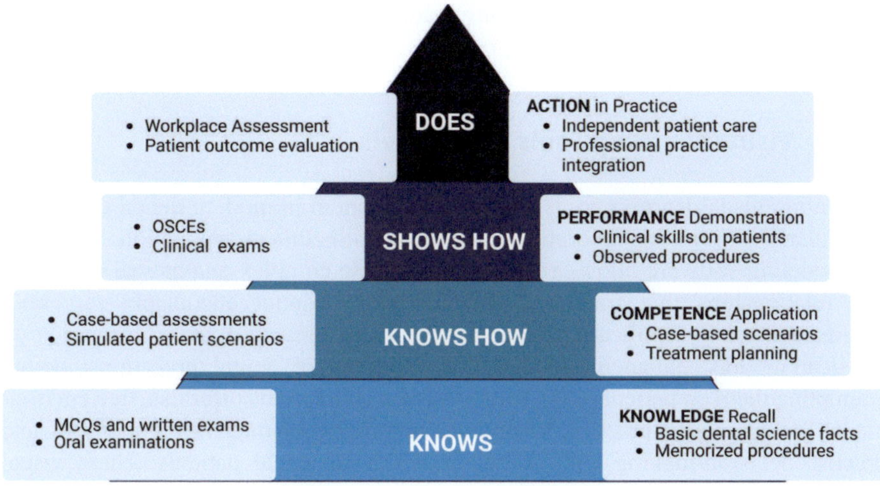

Fig. 2.2 *Miller's Pyramid* for clinical competence in dental education—progression from knowledge to clinical practice in dental education

completion times or qualitative assessment using standardised rubrics, enabling objective evaluation of student performance against established standards [13].

The **achievability** criterion demands careful calibration of objectives to students' current skill levels, available resources and allocated instructional time, recognising that whilst objectives should present meaningful challenges to promote growth, setting unrealistic expectations undermines student motivation and may result in superficial learning. Educational objectives gain relevance when they connect to the dental programme's broader goals and the authentic challenges graduates will face in clinical practice—making explicit how each learning outcome contributes to developing competent practitioners who can meet contemporary oral healthcare needs. The **time-bound dimension** introduces accountability by establishing specific timeframes for achievement—whether by the end of a lecture, a clinical session, a course or a programme year—creating natural assessment points and helping faculty and students manage learning progression effectively.

The exemplar SMART objective for periodontics—'By the end of the third-year periodontics course, students will be able to perform scaling and root planing on a patient with moderate periodontitis, achieving at least 90% plaque removal as verified by a clinical instructor'—demonstrates how these criteria work together to create a comprehensive learning target. It specifically identifies the procedural skill (scaling and root planing), the clinical context (moderate periodontitis), measurable success criteria (90% plaque removal), verification method (instructor assessment), and achievable skill level appropriate for third-year students, relevance to essential periodontal therapy competencies and a clear timeframe (course completion). Such meticulously constructed objectives form the cornerstone of effective dental education, providing clear direction for curriculum design, instructional strategies and assessment methodologies and ensuring graduates possess the comprehensive competencies required for professional practice.

2.2.5 Visual Learning Tools and Models

Integrating visual learning tools has become essential in modern dental education, particularly for bridging theoretical knowledge with clinical application. Advanced 3D modeling software allows students to visualise complex anatomical structures and relationships that traditional 2D textbooks cannot adequately represent. Augmented reality applications enable students to overlay digital information on physical models, enhancing spatial understanding of dental procedures before attempting them on patients [14]. Virtual patient simulations offer risk-free environments for diagnostic practice, where students can encounter rare conditions and practise decision-making without consequences to actual patients. These visual tools are particularly valuable in resource-constrained settings where patient exposure may be limited, as they can partially compensate for gaps in clinical experience whilst standardising educational exposure across diverse institutional settings [15]. Faculty should strategically incorporate these tools as supplements to, rather than replacements for, hands-on experience, using them to prepare students for clinical encounters, reinforce learning after practical sessions and provide remediation for students requiring additional practise in specific competency areas.

2.3 Educational Goals: National and Institutional Perspectives

2.3.1 Dental Council of India (DCI) Competency Framework

The Dental Council of India (DCI) has developed a comprehensive Competency-Based Dental Education (CBDE) framework that serves as the foundation for dental education throughout India. This framework represents a shift from traditional knowledge-based curricula toward an outcomes-focused approach that prioritises the development of specific competencies essential for effective dental practice. At its core, the DCI competency framework is organised into five interconnected domains that collectively define the modern dental professional. The Professionalism domain emphasises the importance of ethical conduct, personal integrity and respect for patients—establishing the moral foundation upon which all clinical practice rests. The communication and collaboration domain recognises that effective dental care extends beyond technical skills, including communicating clearly with patients, working productively with colleagues and collaborating across healthcare disciplines [16].

The patient care domain forms the clinical centre of the framework, encompassing the comprehensive cycle of diagnosis, treatment planning, intervention and prevention. This is complemented by the practice management domain, which acknowledges that dental professionals must develop business acumen and organisational skills to deliver care efficiently within various practice settings (Fig. 2.3). Finally, the critical thinking and research domain reflects the profession's commitment to evidence-based practice and continuous advancement through scientific inquiry. Through this structured framework, the DCI ensures dental graduates possess the technical competence to perform procedures and the professional attributes, communication skills, business understanding and critical thinking abilities necessary to provide holistic oral healthcare in today's complex healthcare environment [17].

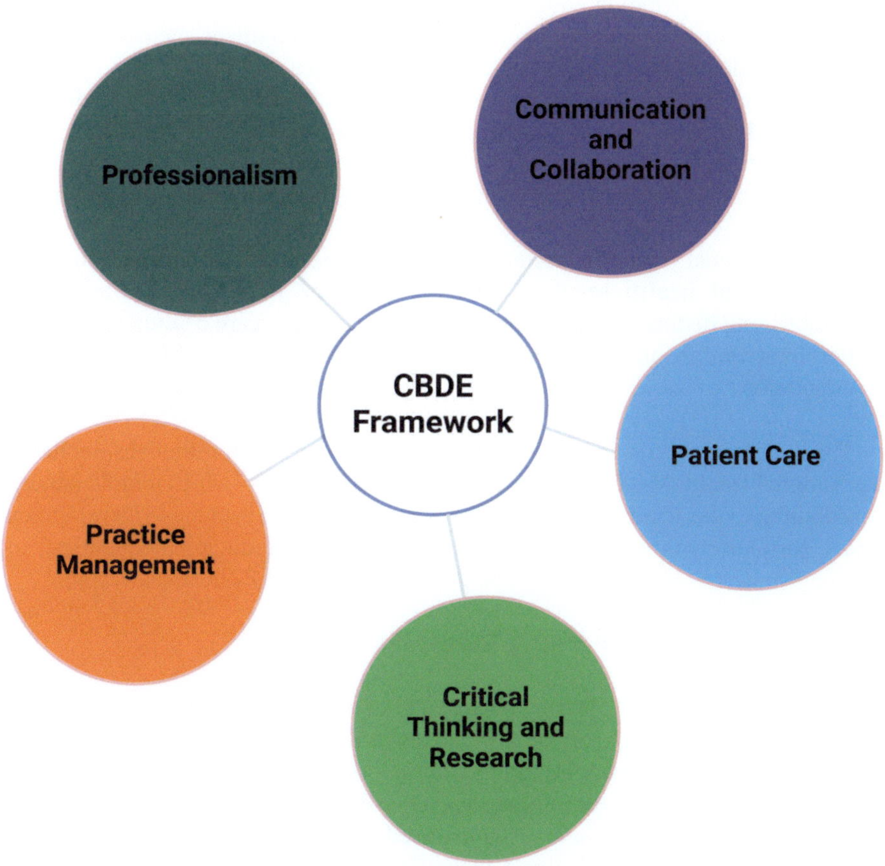

Fig. 2.3 The CBDE framework—the competency-based dental education (CBDE) framework comprises five interconnected domains centred on a core foundation

2.3.2 Overarching National Goals for Dental Workforce Development

2.3.2.1 Strategic Goals for Addressing India's Oral Health Challenges

India faces substantial oral healthcare challenges that require coordinated national action. The government has established four interconnected strategic goals to develop a dental workforce to meet these challenges effectively [18].

- The first goal addresses **dental care access's** quantitative and geographical dimensions. By expanding dental education capacity and implementing targeted incentives for practice in rural and underserved regions, the government aims to correct the current urban concentration of dental professionals and ensure more equitable access nationwide.
- The second goal centres on enhancing **educational quality** through strengthening the competency-based framework established by the Dental Council of India. This includes upgrading educational infrastructure, improving faculty development programmes and implementing rigorous assessment methodologies to ensure graduates possess all necessary competencies.
- The third goal recognises the critical importance of **prevention in reducing disease burden**. Through comprehensive national awareness campaigns and educational initiatives, the government seeks to improve public knowledge of oral hygiene practices and preventive care—reducing the incidence of common oral diseases.
- The fourth goal represents a fundamental shift in **healthcare delivery by integrating oral health services into the primary healthcare** infrastructure. Establishing dedicated oral health units within primary care centres enables earlier intervention and more accessible basic dental services for the general population.

These strategic goals are fully aligned with broader health initiatives, including the National Health Mission and Ayushman Bharat scheme—whilst simultaneously contributing to the achievement of several United Nations Sustainable Development Goals, particularly those related to health, education and reducing inequalities.

2.3.3 Global Benchmarking Examples

Successful adaptations of international dental education models to the Indian context demonstrate how global best practices can be effectively localised whilst respecting resource constraints and cultural considerations. The integration of objective structured clinical examinations (OSCEs) in a few institutions exemplifies the successful implementation of standardised clinical assessment methodologies, modifying station complexity and technology requirements to match available resources whilst maintaining assessment validity [19]. The adaptation of problem-based learning at a few dental colleges in India illustrates thoughtful cultural contextualisation by developing case scenarios reflecting local disease patterns, socioeconomic realities and healthcare delivery challenges. The strategic technology integration into digital dentistry represents employing a tiered approach where students progress from digital case discussions to simulation software and hands-on experience with advanced equipment through industry partnerships that overcome institutional resource limitations [20]. Community-based dental education programmes at KLE Dental College have successfully applied international service-learning models to Indian rural settings, developing structured learning experiences that simultaneously address community needs and student competency development. These exemplars demonstrate that successful global benchmarking requires thoughtful, contextual adaptation rather than directly importing international models.

2.3.4 Institutional Mission and Vision Indian Dental Education

Dental colleges and universities across India establish distinct mission and vision statements that reflect their unique institutional identities whilst addressing common educational priorities (Fig. 2.4). These foundational statements serve as guiding principles for strategic planning, resource allocation and programme development [21, 22].

Excellence in Dental Education Academic excellence forms the cornerstone of most institutional missions. This encompasses curriculum quality, faculty expertise, technological resources and pedagogical approaches. Institutions typically emphasise competency-based education that prepares graduates for clinical practice through comprehensive theoretical knowledge and hands-on clinical experience.

Patient-Centered Care Institutions consistently prioritise the development of patient-centred care approaches. This includes fostering empathy, cultural sensitivity and ethical decision-making abilities. The mission statements often emphasise treating patients as individuals with unique needs rather than focusing solely on procedural competence.

Community Engagement Community service represents a significant commitment for dental institutions. This manifests through outreach programmes, dental camps in underserved areas, public education initiatives and partnerships with local organisations. These activities simultaneously address community needs whilst providing students with valuable clinical and social experiences.

Research and Innovation Research advancement appears prominently in institutional missions, reflecting the profession's commitment to evidence-based practice. Institutions support research through dedicated facilities, faculty development,

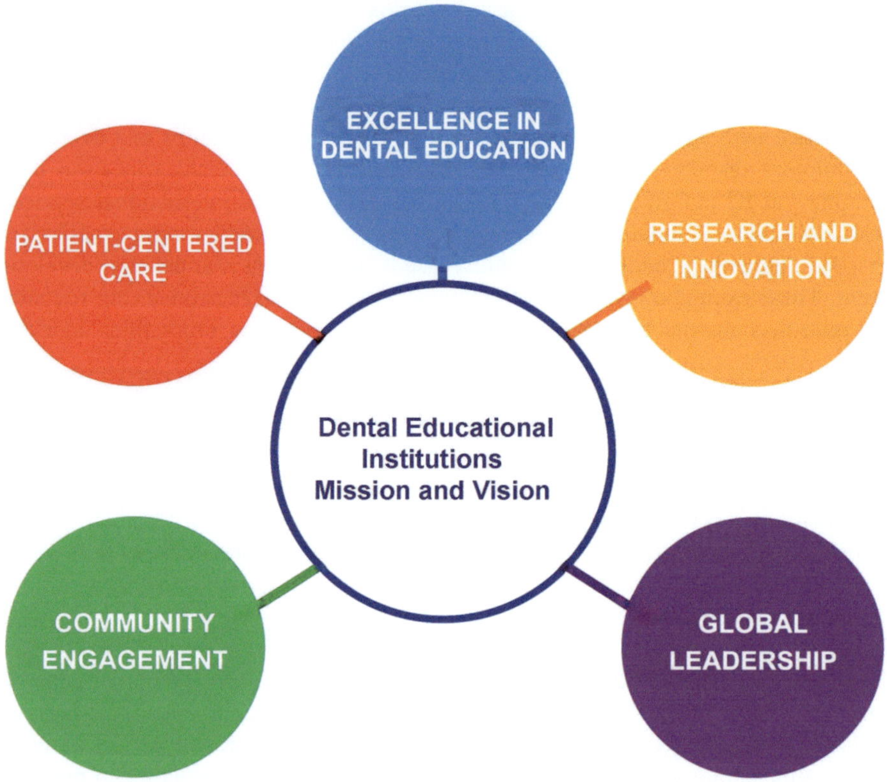

Fig. 2.4 Institutional mission and vision in Indian dental education

student research opportunities and partnerships with other academic and healthcare organisations.

Global Leadership Many institutions aspire to leadership positions within dental education. This ambition drives quality improvement initiatives, international collaborations and adherence to global best practices. Institutions may pursue international accreditation, faculty exchanges and global partnerships to strengthen their reputation and educational offerings.

These mission elements collectively shape institutional culture and educational approaches, providing direction for all stakeholders whilst maintaining alignment with national workforce development goals and regulatory requirements.

2.3.5 Specific Institutional Goals

2.3.5.1 Research

The College of Dentistry is committed to advancing oral health knowledge through robust research initiatives. We are establishing dedicated research centres focusing on critical areas—including oral cancer, implantology and regenerative dentistry—to drive innovation in dental care. Our faculty and students are encouraged to engage in meaningful research activities and publish their findings in respected peer-reviewed journals, contributing to the global body of dental knowledge. Through strategic collaborations with other academic institutions and industry partners, we conduct translational research that bridges the gap between laboratory discoveries and clinical applications—ultimately leading to new treatments and technologies that improve patient outcomes.

2.3.5.2 Community Outreach

Our commitment to community service is demonstrated through comprehensive outreach programmes addressing oral health disparities. We regularly organise dental camps and mobile clinics in underserved areas, providing essential free or low-cost dental care to vulnerable populations without access to these services. We have established strong partnerships with local schools and community organisations to promote oral health education and prevention strategies—empowering communities with knowledge for better oral health. Additionally, our dental students receive training in community-based participatory research, equipping them with the skills to identify and address oral health disparities through evidence-based approaches that respect community needs and contexts.

2.3.5.3 Specialised Training Programmes

The college offers advanced educational opportunities through comprehensive specialised training programmes that prepare dental professionals for the evolving demands of modern dentistry. Our postgraduate and continuing dental education programmes cover specialized areas—including orthodontics, endodontics and oral and maxillofacial surgery—allowing practitioners to develop expertise in their chosen fields. We have developed innovative fellowship programmes that train dental professionals in cutting-edge techniques and technologies—ensuring they remain at the forefront of dental innovation. Through collaborations with prestigious international institutions, we provide exchange programmes and global learning opportunities that expose our students to diverse dental practices and cultural perspectives—enhancing their ability to serve in an increasingly interconnected world.

2.3.6 Institutional Assessment and Continuous Quality Improvement

Dental institutions maintain educational excellence through systematic assessment and continuous quality improvement (CQI). This comprehensive approach ensures institutions remain responsive to evolving healthcare needs and academic standards (Fig. 2.5).

The foundation of effective CQI begins with rigorous self-study and evaluation. Institutions conduct regular internal assessments to identify organisational strengths and weaknesses, educational effectiveness and potential areas for enhancement. This critical self-examination provides the basis for targeted improvement initiatives. External accreditation is an essential validation mechanism, offering an objective assessment of institutional quality against established standards. Accreditation processes typically involve comprehensive curriculum reviews, faculty qualifications, facilities, student outcomes and administrative processes by recognised bodies such as the Dental Council of India.

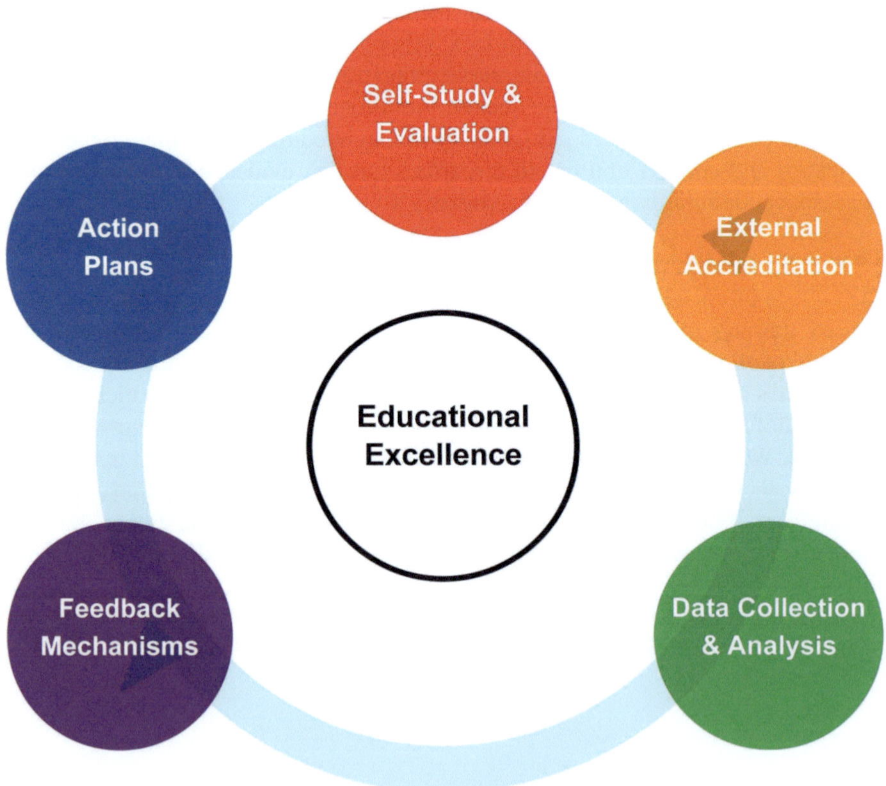

Fig. 2.5 Continuous quality improvement (CQI) framework for dental education excellence

Data collection and analysis form the empirical foundation of the CQI process. Institutions systematically gather and analyse relevant metrics, including student performance data, graduate outcomes, faculty development activities and patient care statistics. This evidence-based approach enables institutions to track progress against established benchmarks and identify emerging trends. Comprehensive feedback mechanisms ensure that improvement efforts incorporate perspectives from all stakeholders [23]. This includes formal and informal input from students, faculty, administrators, patients, alumni and employers. Multi-source feedback provides valuable insights into the practical effectiveness of educational programmes and identifies potential blind spots in institutional self-assessment. The CQI cycle culminates in the development and implementation of structured action plans. These plans translate assessment findings into concrete improvement strategies with clear timelines, responsible parties and measurable outcomes. Practical action plans prioritise interventions based on their potential impact and feasibility.

2.4 Formulating Educational Goals and Objectives for BDS Programmes

2.4.1 Alignment with National Health Priorities

The educational goals for Bachelor of Dental Surgery (BDS) programmes in India must be strategically aligned with the nation's pressing health priorities to ensure graduates can effectively address the country's oral health challenges. Addressing the high prevalence of dental caries and periodontal disease should be central to the curriculum, equipping students with specialised knowledge in prevention, early diagnosis and cost-effective interventions suitable for widespread implementation across diverse populations [16]. Similarly, tackling oral cancer—a significant public health concern in India with higher incidence rates than many other countries—necessitates robust educational components focusing on risk factor identification, screening methodologies and community-based preventive approaches. Improving oral health literacy across diverse socioeconomic groups represents another crucial educational goal, preparing students to develop and implement educational campaigns and communication strategies tailored to different population segments with varying literacy levels and cultural backgrounds. Furthermore, BDS programmes must prepare graduates for the realities of providing care in resource-limited settings, emphasising innovative approaches, preventive strategies and appropriate technology solutions that work effectively within constraints typical of rural and underserved communities [24]. Finally, these educational goals should emphasise integrating oral health with general health initiatives, fostering interprofessional education and collaborative practice models that acknowledge the bidirectional relationship between oral health and systemic conditions such as diabetes, cardiovascular disease and pregnancy outcomes.

2.4.2 Integration with Cultural and Socioeconomic Contexts

The formulation of educational goals for dental programmes in India must be deeply rooted in the country's unique cultural and socioeconomic landscape to ensure the relevance and effectiveness of graduates in their professional practice. Developing cultural competence represents a fundamental educational goal. It requires systematic exposure to and understanding of India's diverse linguistic, religious and regional communities and their health beliefs, dietary practices and unique oral health challenges [16]. Addressing the stark oral health disparities between urban and rural populations demands educational approaches that sensitize students to these inequities whilst building their capacity to develop targeted interventions for disadvantaged communities through rural postings, community outreach programmes and public health dentistry training. The curriculum should also intentionally incorporate knowledge of traditional practices affecting oral health, including beneficial conventional oral hygiene methods and potentially harmful practices, enabling graduates to engage with these cultural realities whilst promoting evidence-based care respectfully [25]. Preparing students to work effectively within India's complex mixed healthcare delivery system, government facilities, corporate hospitals, private practices and charitable institutions requires educational goals to understand healthcare financing, insurance systems and operational models across these diverse settings. Additionally, fostering awareness of affordability considerations in treatment planning constitutes an essential educational goal, ensuring graduates can balance clinical excellence with economic realities by developing skills in providing a spectrum of treatment options at varying price points without compromising quality of care.

2.4.3 Ethics and Professional Identity Formation

Professional identity formation in dental education requires intentional developmental scaffolding beyond traditional ethics coursework—creating a systematic progression from knowledge acquisition to values internalisation throughout the curriculum. Early foundations in the pre-clinical years should establish theoretical ethical frameworks through case-based discussions addressing fundamental principles, including autonomy, beneficence and justice, whilst initiating socialisation through white coat ceremonies, professional oaths and early clinic observations that introduce professional norms and responsibilities [26]. Clinical transition phases should implement structured ethical reasoning exercises connecting theoretical concepts to practical decisions, with guided reflection protocols helping students process challenging patient interactions, conflicting values and emotional responses to clinical situations. Advanced identity consolidation in the final programme stages should incorporate progressive professional responsibility, supervised ethical decision-making in complex cases and interprofessional ethics discussions that prepare students for practice realities. Faculty role modeling represents the most potent influence on identity formation, requiring explicit attention to the 'hidden curriculum'—through faculty development in mindful practice, ethical teaching behaviours and constructive approaches to addressing lapses in professional conduct [27]. Assessment of professional identity development must move beyond knowledge testing to include multisource feedback, reflective portfolio assessment and longitudinal observation of professional behaviours in increasingly complex situations that reveal values internalisation rather than mere compliance with external expectations.

2.4.4 Balancing Global Standards with Local Needs

Indian dental education faces the complex challenge of maintaining a delicate balance between international benchmarks and context-specific requirements, necessitating thoughtfully crafted educational goals. Adhering to globally recognised standards of dental education represents a foundational goal, ensuring Indian graduates possess core competencies consistent with international norms in biomedical sciences, clinical skills, professional ethics and evidence-based practice—thereby facilitating global mobility and recognition of Indian dental qualifications [4]. Simultaneously, educational goals must prioritise adapting international best practices to local contexts, encouraging critical evaluation of worldwide evidence and techniques through the lens of Indian epidemiological patterns, healthcare infrastructure limitations and cultural appropriateness to develop contextually relevant applications. The curriculum should prepare graduates for Indian and international practice opportunities through educational goals that develop universal clinical excellence whilst incorporating specific competencies required for Indian licensure and those valued in global settings—including advanced technology proficiency and research capabilities [28]. Developing context-specific solutions for uniquely Indian oral health challenges constitutes another critical educational goal, fostering problem-solving skills focused on issues relevant to the Indian population, such as tobacco-related oral lesions, paediatric malnutrition impacts on oral health and oral manifestations of tropical diseases [29]. Finally, educational goals should emphasise fostering innovation appropriate for the Indian healthcare infrastructure and stimulating creativity in developing affordable diagnostic tools, preventive strategies and treatment methodologies suited to low-resource settings through project-based learning, innovation competitions and collaboration with engineering and public health disciplines.

2.4.5 Interprofessional Education Opportunities

Strategic integration of interprofessional education (IPE) experiences throughout the dental curriculum prepares graduates for collaborative practice realities whilst enhancing their understanding of dentistry's role within broader healthcare systems. Early exposure through common foundational courses in basic sciences, ethics and healthcare systems—with medical, nursing and allied health students—establishes shared knowledge foundations whilst fostering recognition of complementary roles before professional identities become rigidly established [30]. Case-based learning scenarios addressing complex patient needs requiring multidisciplinary approaches—such as diabetes management, maxillofacial trauma, or geriatric care—develop collaborative reasoning skills through facilitated small-group discussions where each profession contributes its unique perspective to comprehensive care planning. Clinical interprofessional experiences should progress from observation of collaborative care models to participation in team-based clinics where dental students work alongside other health professions students under the supervision of faculty from respective disciplines [31]. Community-based interprofessional projects addressing population health needs strengthen teamwork capabilities whilst developing shared commitment to addressing healthcare disparities. Implementation within the Indian context requires creative scheduling solutions—acknowledging different academic calendars across health professions—developing faculty skilled in interprofessional facilitation and institutional structures supporting collaboration across traditionally siloed departments or even separate colleges within university systems.

2.4.6 Curriculum Mapping

Curriculum mapping documents the relationship between course objectives, programme goals and professional competencies, ensuring that all essential competencies are addressed throughout the curriculum whilst helping to identify gaps or redundancies [32]. Effective curriculum mapping in dental education involves identifying the competencies required for the dental practice, mapping these competencies to specific courses and learning activities, ensuring a logical progression of learning from basic to complex skills, integrating pre-clinical and clinical experiences and regularly reviewing and updating the curriculum map to reflect changes in the profession and educational goals [33]. A well-designed curriculum map helps dental educators ensure that their programme provides students with the knowledge, skills and attitudes needed for successful dental practice in the Indian context.

2.4.7 Student Engagement Strategies

Fostering meaningful student engagement in dental education requires multifaceted approaches that address the cognitive, emotional and social dimensions of learning. Problem-based learning scenarios derived from authentic Indian clinical contexts create relevance whilst challenging students to apply theoretical knowledge to practical situations they will encounter in practice [34]. Strategically implemented peer teaching opportunities, where senior students guide juniors through procedures or concepts they have mastered, build teaching competencies in advanced students whilst providing near-peer learning advantages for juniors. Gamification elements—including achievement badges for clinical milestones, leaderboards for academic performance and simulation competitions—can transform routine skill development into motivating challenges that stimulate continued effort. Community engagement projects connecting coursework to real public health needs create purpose-driven learning whilst developing social responsibility. Technology-enhanced active learning using audience response systems, collaborative digital platforms and learning management systems can transform traditionally passive learning experiences into interactive sessions that maintain attention and improve knowledge retention [35]. Implementation of these engagement strategies must be calibrated to student readiness, progressively increasing autonomy as students develop self-regulation skills throughout the curriculum.

2.5 Implementation Across the BDS Curriculum

2.5.1 First Year BDS

The first year of the Bachelor of Dental Surgery (BDS) curriculum is the critical foundation for the entire professional education—strategically focusing on basic sciences whilst introducing students to the dental profession's fundamental concepts. During this formative period, educational objectives predominantly address the cognitive domain, establishing essential knowledge frameworks whilst initiating the preliminary development of psychomotor skills that will later evolve into clinical competencies. Human anatomy, physiology and biochemistry relevant to dental practice constitute core knowledge areas, providing students with a comprehensive understanding of structural and functional human biology—with particular emphasis on head and neck anatomy, oral cavity structures and biochemical processes relevant to oral health and disease. Dental anatomy and oral histology studies develop specialised knowledge of tooth morphology, development patterns and microscopic structures of oral tissues, creating the foundation for understanding normal versus pathological conditions in future clinical contexts. Introducing basic dental materials and their properties familiarises students with the scientific principles underlying materials used in dental procedures—including their composition, manipulation characteristics and appropriate applications for different clinical scenarios.

Beyond scientific knowledge, first-year objectives include an introduction to dental ethics and professionalism, initiating students' professional identity formation by exploring core values, ethical principles and patient-centred care philosophies that will guide their careers. The critical development of manual dexterity through preclinical exercises begins the systematic building of psychomotor skills through carefully designed activities that progressively advance hand-eye coordination, spatial perception and fine motor control necessary for future clinical procedures. Example objectives such as 'Identify and describe the histological features of oral tissues' establish clear cognitive expectations for microscopic identification skills. At the same time, 'Demonstrate proper handling of basic dental instruments' begins building fundamental psychomotor abilities through specific, observable behaviours. The integrative objective to 'Explain the relevance of basic sciences to clinical dental practice' fosters meaningful connections between theoretical knowledge and future clinical applications, preventing compartmentalisation of learning and establishing patterns of integrative thinking essential for practical clinical reasoning in subsequent years.

2.5.2 Second Year BDS

The second year of the BDS curriculum represents a strategic bridge between foundational sciences and clinical applications, building upon first-year knowledge whilst progressively shifting toward dental-specific domains and introducing increasingly complex psychomotor and affective objectives. This transition year deepens discipline-specific knowledge through focused study of dental pathology and microbiology, where students develop a comprehensive understanding of oral disease processes, microbial etiology and pathogenesis mechanisms that underlie conditions they will diagnose and treat in clinical settings. Pharmacology relevant to dental practice introduces students to therapeutic agents commonly used in dentistry, including local anaesthetics, analgesics, antibiotics and anxiety management medications—emphasising mechanisms of action, dosing considerations and potential adverse effects or interactions. Preclinical training in restorative dentistry and prosthodontics forms the cornerstone of psychomotor skill development during this period, with students practicing cavity preparations, restoration techniques and prosthetic procedures on dental simulators and phantom heads before patient contact.

Introducing clinical diagnosis and treatment planning initiates students into diagnostic reasoning processes through case-based learning, simulated patient scenarios and observational experiences that develop systematic patient assessment and care planning approaches. Developing communication skills for patient interaction introduces crucial affective domain competencies, with students learning and practising effective interview techniques, empathic responses and straightforward explanation methods that will form the foundation of their therapeutic relationships. Example objectives such as "Diagnose common oral pathological conditions from clinical presentations' demonstrate the increasing cognitive complexity expected at this level, requiring application and analysis rather than mere recall. The psychomotor objective, 'Perform basic dental procedures on phantom heads', establishes clear performance expectations for skill development in a controlled environment. In contrast, the integrative objective 'Correlate clinical findings with underlying pathophysiological processes', fosters the clinically relevant connections between observed manifestations and disease mechanisms, developing the causal reasoning essential for practical diagnostic thinking and treatment planning in subsequent clinical years.

2.5.3 Third Year BDS

The third year marks a transformative transition from preclinical simulation to supervised clinical practice, with educational objectives increasingly emphasising integrating knowledge, skills and professional attitudes in authentic patient care contexts. This pivotal year focuses on comprehensive oral diagnosis and treatment planning competencies, developing students' abilities to gather, interpret and synthesise patient information from multiple sources to formulate evidence-based, patient-centred treatment approaches across various common dental conditions. Basic clinical procedures in different dental specialties constitute the core psychomotor development area, with students performing fundamental procedures in restorative dentistry, endodontics, periodontics and prosthodontics under close faculty supervision, progressively advancing from simple to moderately complex interventions as competence develops. Training in oral medicine and radiology enhances diagnostic capabilities through specialised knowledge of oral manifestations of systemic diseases, principles of radiographic interpretation and appropriate use of diagnostic imaging modalities, developing crucial skills for identifying dental and non-dental pathologies.

Periodontics and conservation dentistry receive particular emphasis this year, with students developing competence in non-surgical periodontal therapy and direct restorative procedures that constitute most of the general dental practice. The introduction to public health dentistry broadens students' perspectives beyond individual patient care to population-based approaches, epidemiological principles and preventive strategies applicable to community settings. Example objectives such as 'Perform basic periodontal treatment under supervision' clearly delineate expected clinical competencies with appropriate supervision levels. At the same time, 'Developing treatment plans addressing multiple dental needs' requires higher-order cognitive skills, including analysis, synthesis and evaluation. The preventive focus of 'Implement preventive strategies for high-risk patients' demonstrates the application of risk assessment concepts to individualised patient care, developing the evidence-based preventive orientation essential for contemporary dental practice. These carefully structured third-year objectives collectively guide the critical transition from theoretical knowledge to clinical application, establishing the framework for increasingly independent patient management in the final year.

2.5.4 Final Year BDS

The final year of the BDS curriculum represents the culmination of progressive skill development, focusing on consolidating clinical competence across all dental specialties whilst preparing students for the transition to independent professional practice. Educational objectives at this advanced stage emphasise higher-level cognitive functions, including clinical decision-making, critical analysis of complex cases, evidence-based practice integration and refinement of complex psychomotor skills and full embodiment of professional values. Advanced clinical procedures in all dental specialties form the core focus, with students performing increasingly complex interventions including multi-surface restorations, complete and partial dentures, endodontic treatments and minor oral surgical procedures with decreasing levels of direct supervision as competence develops. Comprehensive patient management abilities expand beyond individual procedures to managing complete treatment sequences for patients with multiple interrelated dental problems, developing crucial case management skills for future practice contexts.

Oral and maxillofacial surgery training advances surgical competencies by performing extractions of increasing complexity, managing surgical complications and exposure to advanced procedures performed by specialists, developing technical skills and appropriate referral judgment. Paediatric dentistry and orthodontics receive dedicated focus, with students developing specialised approaches for managing child patients, performing age-appropriate preventive and restorative procedures and identifying orthodontic issues requiring intervention or referral. Practice management and legal aspects of dentistry prepare students for the business and regulatory dimensions of professional practice, introducing concepts of practice organisation, financial management, quality assurance and compliance with legal and regulatory requirements. Example objectives such as 'Manage patients with complex dental needs independently' clearly establish expectations for increasing clinical autonomy appropriate to final-year status. At the same time, 'Apply evidence-based approaches to clinical decision-making' emphasises the integration of current scientific evidence with clinical expertise and patient preferences. The comprehensive objective, 'Demonstrate proficiency in all core clinical procedures', establishes clear expectations for achieving entry-level competence across the full spectrum of general dental procedures before graduation, ensuring graduates are prepared for professional practice responsibilities.

2.5.5 Internship

The culminating internship year provides an invaluable structured transition between supervised education and independent practice, with educational objectives focused on consolidating clinical competence, developing practice efficiency and solidifying professional identity in authentic practice environments. Rotations through various dental specialties expose interns to advanced procedures and specialised patient management approaches, developing both referral judgment and expanded clinical capabilities in areas of personal interest. Community-based practice experiences place interns in diverse settings including rural clinics, school-based programmes and public health departments, developing adaptability to different practice models, resource levels and patient populations whilst fostering social responsibility and understanding of healthcare disparities. Emergency dental care rotations develop crucial competencies in rapid assessment, pain management and definitive or temporary intervention for acute dental conditions, preparing graduates for managing unscheduled emergencies in future practice settings.

Interdisciplinary collaboration opportunities develop team-based care competencies through interactions with other healthcare professionals, including physicians, nurses and allied dental personnel, fostering an understanding of integrated healthcare approaches and effective communication across disciplinary boundaries [36]. Preparation for professional licensure includes structured reviews of examination content, mock clinical assessments and guidance on regulatory requirements for practice establishment, ensuring graduates can successfully navigate the transition to licensed professional status. Example objectives such as 'Manage a full patient load efficiently and effectively' emphasise developing practice efficiency and time management skills essential for sustainable professional practice. In contrast, 'Adapt clinical skills to resource-constrained settings' develops flexibility and innovation in applying clinical knowledge across diverse practice contexts. The collaborative objective 'Collaborate effectively with other healthcare professionals' recognises the increasingly interprofessional nature of contemporary healthcare, preparing graduates for integrated practice models that optimise patient outcomes through coordinated care approaches. These carefully designed internship objectives ensure that BDS graduates emerge with technical competence and the comprehensive professional capabilities needed for successful, ethical, patient-centred dental practice.

2.6 Assessment of Educational Goals and Objectives

2.6.1 Integrated Assessment Framework

A comprehensive assessment system in dental education must align with educational objectives across all domains of learning [37, 38]:

2.6.1.1 Written Assessments for Cognitive Domain

A well-designed assessment system in dental education must comprehensively evaluate student performance across all learning domains whilst maintaining alignment with established educational objectives. The cognitive domain assessment component employs various written formats to measure knowledge acquisition and application levels [39].

Multiple-choice questions are an efficient evaluation tool for assessing the breadth of knowledge across foundational sciences and clinical principles. This format allows educators to sample various content areas time-efficiently, making it particularly valuable for comprehensive examinations. These questions can be designed with varying complexity to assess different cognitive levels, from basic recall to application of principles [40].

Short answer questions require students to synthesise information and articulate key concepts concisely. This format evaluates both content knowledge and the ability to organise thoughts coherently. Students must demonstrate understanding without the recognition cues in multiple-choice formats, providing a more authentic assessment of mastery of knowledge [41, 42].

Essay questions assess higher-order cognitive skills, including analysis, synthesis and evaluation. This format allows students to demonstrate complex reasoning, integrate multiple concepts and develop well-supported arguments [43]. Essays are particularly valuable for evaluating critical thinking and the ability to address multifaceted problems in dental practice.

Case-based questions contextualise assessment within authentic clinical scenarios, bridging theoretical knowledge and practical application. These questions present students with patient situations that mirror actual practice, requiring them to analyse presented information, formulate differential diagnoses, propose evidence-based treatment plans and justify clinical decisions [44].

These complementary assessment methods comprehensively evaluate cognitive competencies, ensuring dental graduates possess the foundational knowledge and analytical skills required for effective clinical practice. The selection and balance of these methods should align with specific learning objectives and the developmental stage of the students being assessed (Fig. 2.6).

This illustration presents a structured overview of assessment methodologies in dental education, organised by domains (cognitive, psychomotor and affective) and approaches (formative and summative).

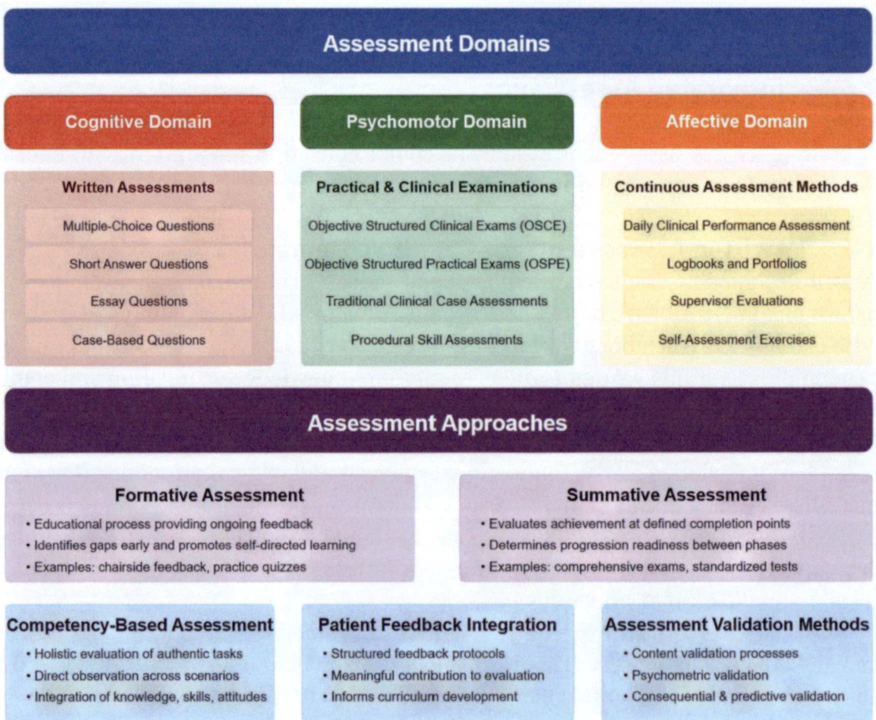

Fig. 2.6 Comprehensive framework for dental education assessment methods

2.6.1.2 Practical and Clinical Examinations for Psychomotor Domain

The comprehensive assessment of dental students' psychomotor skills requires multiple complementary approaches to evaluate technical proficiency across various clinical contexts. Four primary assessment methodologies work in concert to provide a complete picture of students' procedural capabilities [45].

Objective structured clinical examinations (OSCEs) provide a standardised approach to evaluating specific clinical competencies. These assessments consist of timed stations where students perform defined tasks or demonstrate particular skills under direct observation [46]. Each station focuses on discrete elements of clinical practice, such as patient history-taking, radiographic interpretation, or specific diagnostic procedures. The standardised format ensures consistent evaluation criteria across all students, enhancing assessment reliability and fairness.

Objective structured practical examinations (OSPEs) apply a similar station-based methodology to assess laboratory procedures and preclinical skills. These examinations evaluate fundamental technical abilities before patient interaction, including dental material handling, cavity preparation [47], prosthodontic procedures and instrument manipulation. OSPEs are critical gatekeepers, ensuring students possess an adequate technical foundation before progressing to clinical patient care.

Traditional clinical case assessments require students to manage actual patients comprehensively, from initial examination through diagnosis, treatment planning, intervention and follow-up care. These evaluations provide the most authentic measurement of integrated clinical competence, as students must synthesise knowledge, technical skills and professional attributes in managing actual patient needs. Faculty evaluate patient care, including diagnostic accuracy, treatment appropriateness, procedural execution and interaction. Procedural skill assessments focus on the technical quality of interventions, evaluating precision, efficiency and adherence to established protocols. These targeted evaluations may include restorative procedures, endodontic treatments, surgical interventions, or prosthodontic fabrication [48]. Assessment criteria typically include preparation design, marginal integrity, functional outcomes and aesthetic results. Together, these assessment methodologies provide a comprehensive evaluation framework for the psychomotor domain, ensuring dental graduates possess the technical proficiency required for safe and effective patient care across all dental disciplines.

2.6.1.3 Continuous Assessment Methods Across Domains

Continuous assessment methodologies play a crucial role in dental education by evaluating student development across cognitive, psychomotor and affective domains. These methods complement summative examinations by offering regular feedback and documenting progression throughout the educational programme.

Daily clinical performance assessment enables real-time evaluation of student-patient interactions in authentic clinical settings. Faculty supervisors observe students during patient care, providing immediate feedback on diagnostic reasoning, treatment execution, communication skills and professional behaviour. This ongoing assessment identifies performance patterns and allows for timely intervention when deficiencies are noted [49]. The immediate nature of this feedback creates valuable learning opportunities at the point of care.

Logbooks and portfolios serve as comprehensive records of students' procedural experience and reflective learning. Students' document clinical cases, laboratory procedures and educational activities whilst reflecting on their experiences and learning outcomes [50]. These tools capture both quantitative data on clinical exposure and qualitative information on professional development. Faculty review these documents periodically to evaluate clinical experience breadth, technical progression and reflective capacity.

Supervisor evaluations provide experienced clinician perspectives on students' multidimensional performance. Clinical faculty assess students across multiple competency domains, including clinical reasoning, technical skills, patient management, professionalism and teamwork. These evaluations often employ standardised rubrics aligned with programme competencies to ensure comprehensive and consistent assessment [51]. Periodic evaluations from multiple supervisors help identify performance trends and development needs.

Self-assessment exercises involve structured reflection on personal performance against established standards. Students evaluate their own strengths, weaknesses and development needs through guided tools that prompt critical analysis of their work. These exercises develop metacognitive skills essential for lifelong professional development whilst fostering accountability for learning outcomes [52]. Faculty review these self-assessments to identify gaps between student perception and external evaluation.

Together, these continuous assessment methods create a comprehensive system for monitoring student development, providing formative feedback and ensuring that students are progressing appropriately toward the competencies required for independent practice.

2.6.2 Formative vs. Summative Assessment

2.6.2.1 Formative Assessment

The BDS curriculum requires thoughtful integration of formative and summative assessment approaches to optimise learning outcomes and ensure graduate competence. Formative assessment functions as an educational process rather than merely an evaluation tool, providing ongoing feedback during skill acquisition and knowledge development phases that guide learning whilst consequences remain low [41, 53]. This continuous feedback mechanism identifies misconceptions, technical errors and performance gaps early in the educational process, enabling timely corrective interventions before deficiencies become entrenched or affect patient care. The approach promotes self-directed learning by helping students recognise their specific development needs and the effectiveness of their study strategies, fostering the reflective practice habits essential for lifelong professional growth [54]. Exemplars of practical formative assessment include daily chairside feedback during clinical procedures, practice quizzes with explanatory answers in introductory science courses and structured peer evaluations of recorded patient interactions, all characterised by their emphasis on improvement rather than grading.

2.6.2.2 Summative Assessment

Summative assessment serves complementary functions within the curriculum, evaluating achievement of educational objectives at defined completion points to ensure students have attained the required competencies before advancing. These assessments determine progression readiness between educational phases including preclinical to clinical transitions, year-to-year advancement and ultimately programme completion and maintaining academic standards and patient safety through evidence-based promotion decisions [31]. Crucially, summative assessments ensure that graduates possess the comprehensive competencies required for independent practice, serving as the profession's quality assurance mechanism for protecting public health. Representative summative assessments include comprehensive university examinations combining written, practical and clinical components; standardized practical tests with defined passing thresholds for critical procedures; and culminating case presentations demonstrating integrated application of knowledge and skills across multiple domains [55]. The effective dental curriculum strategically employs both assessment approaches in a complementary fashion, using formative assessment to optimise learning processes and summative evaluation to verify achievement of required competencies, collectively ensuring graduates possess the knowledge, skills and professional attributes needed for safe, effective dental practice.

2.6.3 Competency-Based Assessment

Competency-based assessment represents a paradigm shift in dental education evaluation, moving beyond isolated knowledge testing towards holistic evaluation of students' abilities to perform authentic professional tasks in realistic contexts. This approach centres on direct observation of clinical skills by qualified faculty evaluators who assess students performing actual dental procedures on patients, using structured rating scales or checklists that capture critical elements of performance, including technical execution, patient management and adherence to safety protocols. These observations occur across multiple patient encounters and varied clinical scenarios, ensuring students consistently demonstrate competence rather than showing isolated successful performances. The assessment of complex problem-solving in realistic contexts forms another cornerstone of the competency-based approach, presenting students with multifaceted clinical scenarios requiring the integration of diagnostic reasoning, treatment planning and technical intervention skills to develop comprehensive solutions for patients with complicated or interdisciplinary needs [12].

The emphasis on integrating knowledge, skills and attitudes distinguish competency-based assessment from traditional compartmentalised evaluation methods, recognising that professional competence emerges from the seamless synthesis of theoretical understanding, technical ability and professional values rather than their independent demonstration. This integration is evaluated through comprehensive patient care experiences where students must simultaneously apply biomedical science concepts, execute technical procedures, communicate effectively and demonstrate professional behaviours within authentic treatment contexts. Multiple assessments over time ensure consistency of performance and developmental progression, with students evaluated repeatedly across varied patients, conditions and contexts throughout their educational programme rather than relying on single-point examinations that might not reflect typical performance or capture improvement trajectories.

Clear performance standards based on professional expectations provide the essential framework for competency assessment, with explicit criteria detailing the specific elements, quality levels and contextual factors that constitute entry-level professional competence [56]. These standards derive from analysis of authentic practice requirements and regulatory expectations for new graduates; ensuring educational assessment aligns directly with the profession's quality standards for patient care. Through this multidimensional, integrated approach to evaluation, competency-based dental education ensures graduates possess not merely isolated knowledge and skills but the comprehensive capability to provide safe, effective patient care in the complex, dynamic dental practice environment.

2.6.4 Patient Feedback Integration

Systematically incorporating patient perspectives into dental education transforms the traditional dyadic teacher-student relationship into a triadic model that honours patients as active participants in the educational process. Structured patient feedback protocols should be implemented across clinical encounters, using validated instruments that assess technical outcomes and communication quality, professionalism and patient-centred care dimensions that faculty supervisors may not fully observe. Patient-derived assessment data should contribute meaningfully to student evaluation through appropriate weighting in competency determinations, particularly for professional attributes and communication skills where patients have unique expertise [57]. Beyond individual assessment, aggregated patient feedback should inform curriculum development through regular analysis, identifying systemic gaps in student preparation, emerging patient expectations and changing care priorities that require curricular adaptation. Patient inclusion on curriculum committees can further institutionalise these perspectives, with representatives from diverse socioeconomic and cultural backgrounds ensuring broad representation of the communities graduates will serve. Ethical implementation requires careful consideration of power dynamics, with clear communication to patients about feedback purposes, confidentiality protections and mechanisms ensuring that participation decisions do not influence care quality [58].

2.6.5 Assessment Validation Methods

Rigorous validation of assessment methods ensures that evaluation practices measure intended learning outcomes rather than unrelated factors or implicit biases [38]. Content validation processes should systematically map assessment items against learning objectives and professional competency frameworks, using expert panels including both subject specialists and assessment methodologists to evaluate relevance, representativeness and comprehensiveness. Psychometric validation must apply appropriate statistical analyses to examination data, including reliability calculations, item analysis and discrimination indices that identify potentially problematic questions or rating scales requiring revision. Consequential validation examines whether assessment practices produce intended educational effects, including appropriate student study behaviours, equitable outcomes across student populations and graduate performance meeting stakeholder expectations. Predictive validation studies tracking the relationship between assessment performance and subsequent clinical competence provide crucial evidence linking educational evaluation to practice readiness. Implementing these validation approaches requires establishing assessment units within dental institutions with appropriate expertise, developing faculty assessment literacy through targeted professional development and creating feedback loops where validation findings drive continuous improvement of evaluation practices [59]. Regular external review by dental education assessment experts further strengthens the validity of evidence whilst identifying potential innovations for enhancing assessment quality.

2.6.6 Sample Assessment Rubrics

Developmentally appropriate assessment rubrics provide concrete tools for evaluating competence progression throughout the dental curriculum. Preclinical procedure rubrics should emphasise foundational elements, including instrument handling, procedural sequencing and basic technical accuracy, with detailed performance level descriptions differentiating between beginning, developing and competent execution of fundamental skills [60]. Early clinical assessment rubrics must address technical proficiency and emergent professional dimensions, including infection control compliance, patient communication, time management and appropriate supervisor engagement, with performance standards calibrated to novice clinician expectations. Advanced clinical rubrics for final-year students should emphasise comprehensive patient management, clinical reasoning quality and adaptive problem-solving during procedural complications and independent professional judgment, with 'competent' standards aligned to entry-level practitioner expectations. Professional behaviour rubrics must span the curriculum with consistent core expectations but progressively increasing standards for self-direction, ethical reasoning sophistication and leadership dimensions as students advance [61]. Implementation requires systematic faculty calibration through regular exercises using video recordings or live demonstrations of varying performance levels, establishing a shared understanding of standards and minimising inter-rater variability [62]. Electronic rubric platforms that capture longitudinal performance data are particularly valuable for tracking developmental progression and identifying students requiring additional support in specific competency domains.

2.7 Challenges and Solutions in Implementation

2.7.1 Resource Limitations and Solutions

2.7.1.1 Infrastructure Challenges

Implementing comprehensive educational objectives in Indian dental education faces significant infrastructural challenges that necessitate creative adaptation and strategic planning to ensure quality outcomes despite resource constraints. The marked variation in facilities across government and private institutions creates educational inequities, with some institutions offering state-of-the-art simulation laboratories, digital radiography and advanced clinical equipment [29]. In contrast, others struggle to maintain basic operational standards for clinical training. This disparity directly impacts the achievement of psychomotor objectives requiring specialised skill development equipment. The limited availability of advanced technological resources, including CAD/CAM systems, cone-beam computed tomography, dental operatory microscopes and digital impression systems, restricts students' exposure to contemporary practice methodologies that are increasingly becoming standard in global dental practice [63]. Additionally, institutions must adapt their educational objectives to available resources without compromising core competency development, requiring careful prioritisation of essential and desirable learning experiences and the development of alternative approaches to achieve similar educational outcomes with different resource configurations.

2.7.1.2 Innovative Solutions

Innovative solutions can substantially mitigate these resource challenges through collaborative and technological approaches. Sharing resources between institutions through formal partnerships and collaborations enables cost-effective access to expensive equipment and specialised facilities, with potential models including regional centres of excellence for specific technical training, cooperative purchasing arrangements for high-cost equipment and exchange programmes allowing students to rotate through differently resourced institutions for comprehensive exposure [64]. Institutions can increasingly utilise technology to overcome physical limitations through virtual simulations, augmented reality training programmes and remote observation of procedures that provide educational exposure to advanced techniques even when physical equipment is unavailable. Dental education programmes must also develop teaching methodologies that achieve objectives with minimal resources, including hybrid models combining limited hands-on experience with extensive pre-procedural simulation, creative use of locally available materials for skill development and adaptation of international educational approaches to resource-constrained settings through locally relevant innovations and simplified procedural protocols that maintain essential quality standards [65].

2.7.1.3 Technology Integration Framework

A structured technology integration framework provides dental institutions at various resource levels with strategic pathways for enhancing education through appropriate digital tools. The foundation level establishes essential digital literacy requirements for all dental programmes regardless of resource availability [66]. These include electronic patient records, basic digital radiography, online learning management systems and fundamental digital communication tools that represent minimum technological competencies for contemporary practice. The intermediate level introduces enhanced educational technologies where resources permit, including simulation systems with haptic feedback, virtual patient cases, CAD design software with limited production capabilities and basic digital workflow exposure in clinical settings. The advanced level incorporates cutting-edge technologies as they become financially accessible, including full digital workflow implementation, AI-assisted diagnostic tools and 3D printing applications and augmented reality surgical planning systems that represent emerging practice standards [67]. This tiered approach enables all institutions to strategically plan technology integration according to available resources whilst establishing clear developmental pathways as additional funding becomes available. Implementation should follow the principle of pedagogical appropriateness, where technology is integrated only when it demonstrably enhances learning outcomes rather than for its novelty, with faculty development preceding each technology introduction to ensure effective educational utilisation [68].

2.7.2 Cultural and Systemic Factors

2.7.2.1 Traditional Learning Approaches

Traditional Learning Approaches: Deeply embedded cultural and systemic factors significantly influence the implementation of contemporary educational approaches in Indian dental education. The historical emphasis on memorisation over critical thinking, reinforced by examination systems that reward recall rather than analysis or application, creates resistance to problem-based learning approaches and hinders the development of the clinical reasoning skills essential for competent patient care [69]. Students often enter dental programmes with limited experience in self-directed learning, having succeeded in educational systems prioritising teacher-centred instruction and prescribed content mastery rather than independent inquiry or personal learning responsibility. This creates challenges when implementing contemporary educational methods requiring greater learner autonomy and initiative [70, 71]. Additionally, hierarchical teacher-student relationships affecting feedback processes can impede the honest communication essential for practical formative assessment, with students hesitant to question authority or admit uncertainty and faculty sometimes interpreting questions as challenges rather than learning opportunities, creating barriers to the open communication required for optimal skill development.

2.7.2.2 Solutions for Cultural Transformation

Effective navigation of these cultural challenges requires thoughtful, incremental approaches to educational transformation. The gradual introduction of active learning methodologies provides a transitional path from traditional to contemporary approaches, beginning with structured activities with clear guidance and explicit expectations before progressing to more open-ended, student-driven learning experiences [72]. Comprehensive faculty development in modern pedagogical approaches is essential, providing instructors with theoretical foundations and practical implementation strategies for student-centred learning, effective questioning techniques, constructive feedback methods and creating psychologically safe learning environments. Institutions must intentionally create a culture valuing inquiry and open communication through modelling by educational leaders, explicit valuing of questions and discussion in assessment systems, creating safe spaces for practice and error without judgment and formal feedback mechanisms that normalise constructive criticism in all directions [73]. These systematic approaches can gradually transform traditional educational cultures into learning communities that foster critical thinking, self-direction and open communication to develop competent, adaptable dental professionals.

2.7.3 Future Directions for Educational Goals and Objectives

2.7.3.1 Emerging Areas for New Objectives

Dental education must continually evolve to incorporate emerging domains shaping the profession's future. Digital dentistry and AI-assisted diagnosis represent transformative areas requiring new educational objectives addressing technical competencies like CAD/CAM restoration design and critical evaluation skills for AI-generated diagnostic suggestions, ensuring graduates can effectively leverage technology whilst maintaining professional judgment [74]. Interdisciplinary collaboration with other healthcare professionals is increasingly essential as oral-systemic health connections become better understood, necessitating objectives focused on team-based care models, effective interprofessional communication and understanding of integrated care pathways for conditions like diabetes and cardiovascular disease that have significant oral health dimensions. Personalized and precision dentistry emerges as another crucial domain, requiring objectives that develop genomic literacy, an understanding of biomarker significance and the ability to tailor treatments based on individual patient characteristics, including genetic predispositions, microbiome profiles and personalised risk assessments [75].

Tele-dentistry for reaching remote populations represents another emerging priority area, requiring educational objectives addressing remote assessment methodologies, digital communication skills and adaptation of clinical decision-making to limited-information contexts to help address persistent access-to-care challenges in underserved regions [76]. Environmental sustainability in dental practice must also be integrated into educational objectives, developing awareness of dentistry's ecological impact and competencies in waste reduction, energy conservation and environmentally responsible material selection that align professional practice with broader societal sustainability goals. These emerging domains will require thoughtful integration into already-dense curricula, potentially necessitating reconsideration of traditional content to create space for these forward-looking competencies.

2.7.3.2 Maintaining Relevance in a Changing Healthcare Landscape

Ensuring the continued relevance of dental education requires systematic curriculum evaluation and adaptation processes. Regularly reviewing and updating goals and objectives should occur through formal cycles incorporating emerging scientific evidence, changing practice patterns, technological innovations and evolving regulatory requirements to prevent educational stagnation. The involvement of diverse stakeholders in curriculum development—including practitioners, specialists, public health experts, patients and students—provides essential perspective diversity that helps identify emerging needs and evaluate existing approaches from multiple viewpoints [77]. Educational programmes must continuously benchmark against global standards whilst maintaining local relevance, adopting international best practices where appropriate and ensuring contextual adaptation to India's unique healthcare challenges, resource availability and cultural considerations. Finally, rigorous research on educational outcomes must inform continuous improvement through systematic collection of performance data, graduate follow-up studies, employer feedback and patient satisfaction metrics that provide evidence about programme effectiveness in preparing competent practitioners [78]. Through these interconnected approaches, Indian dental education can maintain dynamic relevance in an evolving healthcare environment, continuously refining its educational goals and objectives to prepare graduates for the complex, changing landscape of contemporary and future dental practice.

2.7.4 Faculty Development and Training

Comprehensive faculty development is the cornerstone of successful educational reform in dental institutions, requiring systematic programmes that transform subject matter experts into effective educational facilitators. Structured pedagogical training should address contemporary teaching methodologies—including competency-based education, problem-based learning and technology-enhanced instruction—providing theoretical foundations and practical implementation strategies adapted to the Indian dental education context. Clinical teaching workshops should address the unique challenges of chairside instruction, including balancing patient care with student learning, providing constructive real-time feedback and adapting teaching approaches to different learning styles and student readiness levels. Assessment literacy development must ensure that faculty can design, implement and interpret valid assessments that align with stated learning objectives and provide meaningful feedback for student improvement. [16]. Mentorship programmes pairing experienced educators with newer faculty create supportive relationships for ongoing professional development whilst preserving institutional teaching wisdom. Regular educational scholarship opportunities—including action research projects, conference presentations and publication in dental education journals—develop faculty as both consumers and contributors to the evidence base for dental education [79]. These comprehensive faculty development initiatives require institutional commitment through protected time, recognition in promotion processes and the creation of communities of practice where educators can collaboratively solve teaching challenges.

2.7.5 Quality Assurance Mechanisms

Comprehensive quality assurance systems in dental education require multilevel monitoring mechanisms that systematically evaluate alignment between intended, enacted and achieved curricula. Programme-level review committees should conduct regular curriculum mapping audits examining how course objectives, teaching activities and assessment methods align with programme goals and professional competency frameworks, identifying misalignments requiring modification. Course-level quality circles bringing together faculty, students and educational specialists should meet regularly to review achievement data, student feedback and emerging disciplinary developments, generating continuous improvement recommendations with assigned responsibility and implementation timelines [80]. Clinical teaching quality assurance requires additional mechanisms, including systematic clinical faculty calibration through standardised patient exercises, peer observation programmes with structured feedback protocols and regular audit of student clinical experiences, ensuring appropriate case distribution and procedure volume across all required competency domains. External validation through periodic review by dental education experts from other institutions provides a crucial outside perspective on programme quality, whilst graduate outcome tracking—including licensure examination performance, employer satisfaction and practice pattern analysis—provides ultimate validation of educational effectiveness [81]. Technological support through curriculum management software and learning analytics platforms enables more sophisticated quality monitoring by highlighting patterns that may not be apparent through traditional review mechanisms, including achievement gaps across student populations, curriculum sequencing effects and relationships between specific educational experiences and downstream outcomes.

2.8 Conclusion

Educational goals and objectives form the foundation of an effective dental curriculum. In the Indian context, these must be carefully crafted to address the unique challenges and opportunities of the healthcare environment whilst preparing graduates for local and global practice. By developing clear, measurable and contextually appropriate goals and objectives, dental educators can ensure that the substantial investment in dental education translates to improved oral health outcomes for India's diverse population. The journey from establishing broad educational goals to implementing specific learning objectives requires collaboration among regulatory bodies, institutions, faculty and students. It demands a balance between adhering to global standards of dental education and addressing the unique needs of the Indian population. With thoughtful planning, regular evaluation and continuous improvement, Indian dental education can continue to evolve and excel, producing graduates who are competent practitioners, compassionate healers and lifelong learners committed to improving oral health for all.

Conflict of Interest None.

References

1. Mahal AS, Shah N. Implications of the growth of dental education in India. J Dent Educ. 2006;70(8):884–91. https://doi.org/10.1002/j.0022-0337.2006.70.8.tb04155.x.
2. Jaiswal AK, Srinivas P, Suresh S. Dental manpower in India: changing trends since 1920. Int Dent J. 2014;64(4):213–8. https://doi.org/10.1111/idj.12111.
3. Jarni N, Gurr D. A futures perspective on learning and teaching in higher education: an essay on best and next practices. Trends Higher Educ. 2024;3(3):793–811.
4. Elangovan S, Allareddy V, Singh F, Taneja P, Karimbux N. Indian dental education in the new millennium: challenges and opportunities. J Dent Educ. 2010;74(9):1011–6.
5. Gracco A, De Stefani A, Bruno G. Influence of new technology in dental care: a public health perspective. Int J Environ Res Public Health. 2023;20(7) https://doi.org/10.3390/ijerph20075364.
6. Kaplan MA. Using digital technology to enhance medical education and improve the quality of patient care in a changing global healthcare system. In: Bayar Y, Karabetyan L, editors. Economic and social implications of information and communication technologies. Advances in wireless technologies and telecommunication. Hershey: IGI Global; 2023. p. 20–37.
7. Mather H, Bateman H, Taylor J, Vernazza C, Rothwell C, McCracken G, et al. From inputs to outputs: an analysis of the changes to learning outcomes for dental undergraduate education in the UK. Br Dent J. 2022;232(2):101–7. https://doi.org/10.1038/s41415-022-3873-y.
8. Thornhill-Miller B, Camarda A, Mercier M, Burkhardt JM, Morisseau T, Bourgeois-Bougrine S, et al. Creativity, critical thinking, communication, and collaboration: assessment, certification, and promotion of 21st century skills for the future of work and education. J Intelligence. 2023;11(3) https://doi.org/10.3390/jintelligence11030054.
9. Schuler IM, Bach K, Schadlich P, Rabe U. Developing and evaluating a new preclinical curriculum with focus on prevention in dentistry. Dent J (Basel). 2025;13(2) https://doi.org/10.3390/dj13020081.
10. McHarg J, Kay EJ. Designing a dental curriculum for the twenty-first century. Br Dent J. 2009;207(10):493–7. https://doi.org/10.1038/sj.bdj.2009.1011.
11. Williams BW, Byrne PD, Welindt D, Williams MV. Miller's pyramid and core competency assessment: a study in relationship construct validity. J Contin Educ Heal Prof. 2016;36(4):295–9. https://doi.org/10.1097/CEH.0000000000000117.
12. Tonni I, Gadbury-Amyot CC, Govaerts M, Ten Cate O, Davis J, Garcia LT, et al. ADEA-ADEE shaping the future of dental education III: assessment in competency-based dental education: ways forward. J Dent Educ. 2020;84(1):97–104. https://doi.org/10.1002/jdd.12024.

13. Marchini L, Schneider G, Stanford C. Dental school department strategic planning: a department driven approach. J Dent Educ. 2024;88(11):1462–6. https://doi.org/10.1002/jdd.13623.
14. Bevizova K, Falougy HE, Thurzo A, Harsanyi S. Is virtual reality enhancing dental anatomy education? A systematic review and meta-analysis. BMC Med Educ. 2024;24(1):1395. https://doi.org/10.1186/s12909-024-06233-0.
15. Huang G, Reynolds R, Candler C. Virtual patient simulation at U.S. and Canadian medical schools. Acad Med. 2007;82(5)
16. Deshpande AN, Mathur VP, Lele GS, Nirmal L, Saha S, Muthu MS, et al. Identifying needs and preparing for curriculum changes in Indian dental education. Int J Clin Pediatr Dent. 2024;17(7):842–50. https://doi.org/10.5005/jp-journals-10005-2846.
17. Elendu C, Amaechi DC, Okatta AU, Amaechi EC, Elendu TC, Ezeh CP, et al. The impact of simulation-based training in medical education: a review. Medicine (Baltimore). 2024;103(27):e38813. https://doi.org/10.1097/MD.0000000000038813.
18. Dasson Bajaj P, Shenoy R, Davda LS, Mala K, Bajaj G, Rao A, et al. A scoping review exploring oral health inequalities in India: a call for action to reform policy, practice and research. Int J Equity Health. 2023;22(1):242. https://doi.org/10.1186/s12939-023-02056-5.
19. Shahzad A, Saeed MHB, Paiker S. Dental students' concerns regarding OSPE and OSCE: a qualitative feedback for process improvement. BDJ Open. 2017;3(1):17009. https://doi.org/10.1038/bdjopen.2017.9.
20. Tripathi S, Manoharan PS, Nagda S. Developing an instructional module of 'digital dentistry' for undergraduate prosthodontics curriculum. J Oral Biol Craniofac Res. 2024;14(1):44–8. https://doi.org/10.1016/j.jobcr.2023.12.001.
21. Virdi MS. Reforming undergraduate dental education in India: introducing a credits and semester system. J Dent Educ. 2011;75(12):1596–602.
22. Jessani A, Athanasakos A, Kachwinya S. "A life-changing experience and the beginning of a lifelong commitment": experiences and impact of Global Health Community Service-Learning in undergraduate dental curriculum in Canada. BMC Oral Health. 2024;24(1):799. https://doi.org/10.1186/s12903-024-04539-5.
23. Endalamaw A, Khatri RB, Mengistu TS, Erku D, Wolka E, Zewdie A, et al. A scoping review of continuous quality improvement in healthcare system: conceptualization, models and tools, barriers and facilitators, and impact. BMC Health Serv Res. 2024;24(1):487. https://doi.org/10.1186/s12913-024-10828-0.
24. King S, Thaliph A, Laranjo L, Smith BJ, Eberhard J. Oral health literacy, knowledge and perceptions in a socially and culturally diverse population: a mixed methods study. BMC Public Health. 2023;23(1):1446. https://doi.org/10.1186/s12889-023-16381-5.
25. Tadin A, Poljak Guberina R, Domazet J, Gavic L. Oral hygiene practices and Oral health knowledge among students in Split, Croatia. Healthcare (Basel). 2022;10(2) https://doi.org/10.3390/healthcare10020406.
26. Du X, Al Khabuli JOS, Ba Hattab RAS, Daud A, Philip NI, Anweigi L, et al. Development of professional identity among dental students—a qualitative study. J Dent Educ. 2023;87(1):93–100. https://doi.org/10.1002/jdd.13092.
27. Cantaert GR, Pype P, Valcke M, Lauwerier E. Interprofessional identity in health and social care: analysis and synthesis of the assumptions and conceptions in the literature. Int J Environ Res Public Health. 2022;19(22) https://doi.org/10.3390/ijerph192214799.
28. Jacob KS. Medical Council of India's new competency-based curriculum for medical graduates: a critical appraisal. Indian J Psychol Med. 2019;41(3):203–9. https://doi.org/10.4103/IJPSYM.IJPSYM_166_19.
29. Kakde S, Bedi R, Verma M. Oral health inequalities: a call for action to improve oral health in India. Int Dent J. 2013;63(6):324–8. https://doi.org/10.1111/idj.12048.
30. Alqutaibi AY, Rahhal MM, Awad R, Sultan OS, Iesa MAM, Zafar MS, et al. Implementing and evaluating interprofessional education for dental students: a narrative review. Eur J Dent. 2025; https://doi.org/10.1055/s-0045-1804505.

31. Alexander ES, White AA, Varol A, Appel K, Lieneck C. Team- and problem-based learning in health services: a systematic literature review of recent initiatives in the United States. Educ Sci. 2024;14(5):515.
32. Quinonez RB, Danciu T, Ramaswamy V, Murdoch-Kinch CA. Bridging the gap between dental education and clinical practice: the entrustable professional activities model. J Am Dent Assoc. 2023;154(8):687–9. https://doi.org/10.1016/j.adaj.2023.05.009.
33. Lin GSS, Foo JY, Foong CC. Curriculum mapping of a dental materials science course: a reality check and way forward. BMC Med Educ. 2023;23(1):716. https://doi.org/10.1186/s12909-023-04717-z.
34. Al-Madi EM, Celur SL, Nasim M. Effectiveness of PBL methodology in a hybrid dentistry program to enhance students' knowledge and confidence. (a pilot study). BMC Med Educ. 2018;18(1):270 https://doi.org/10.1186/s12909-018-1392-y.
35. Elsheli J, Patrick A, Stokes C. Community-based education programmes in the context of dental education: a scoping review. Eur J Dent Educ. 2024;28(2):576–90. https://doi.org/10.1111/eje.12986.
36. Annamma LM, Varma SR, Abuttayem H, Prasad P, Azim SA, Odah R, et al. Current challenges in dental education- a scoping review. BMC Med Educ. 2024;24(1):1523. https://doi.org/10.1186/s12909-024-06545-1.
37. Gerhard-Szep S, Guntsch A, Pospiech P, Sohnel A, Scheutzel P, Wassmann T, et al. Assessment formats in dental medicine: an overview. GMS. J Med Educ. 2016;33(4):Doc65 https://doi.org/10.3205/zma001064.
38. Bissell V, Dawson LJ. Assessment and feedback in dental education: a journey. Br Dent J. 2022;233(6):499–502. https://doi.org/10.1038/s41415-022-4968-1.
39. Albino JE, Young SK, Neumann LM, Kramer GA, Andrieu SC, Henson L, et al. Assessing dental students' competence: best practice recommendations in the performance assessment literature and investigation of current practices in predoctoral dental education. J Dent Educ. 2008;72(12):1405–35. https://doi.org/10.1002/j.0022-0337.2008.72.12.tb04620.x.
40. Moss E. Multiple choice questions: their value as an assessment tool. Curr Opin Anaesthesiol. 2001;14(6):661–6. https://doi.org/10.1097/00001503-200112000-00011.
41. Haugen HJ, de Lange T. Multiple choice as formative assessment in dental education. Eur J Dent Educ. 2024;28(3):757–69. https://doi.org/10.1111/eje.13002.
42. Putt O, Westacott R, Sam AH, Gurnell M, Brown CA. Using very short answer errors to guide teaching. Clin Teach. 2022;19(2):100–5. https://doi.org/10.1111/tct.13458.
43. Shamim MS, Zaidi SJA, Rehman A. The revival of essay-type questions in medical education: harnessing artificial intelligence and machine learning. J Coll Physicians Surg Pak. 2024;34(5):595–9. https://doi.org/10.29271/jcpsp.2024.05.595.
44. Shigli K, Aswini YB, Fulari D, Sankeshwari B, Huddar D, Vikneshan M. Case-based learning: a study to ascertain the effectiveness in enhancing the knowledge among interns of an Indian dental institute. J Indian Prosthodont Soc. 2017;17(1):29–34. https://doi.org/10.4103/0972-4052.194945.
45. Al-Zain AO, Abdel-Azim AM, Othman HI. Dental students' didactic and psychomotor skills performance in dental anatomy and preclinical operative dentistry courses in a Saudi governmental school. Int J Dent. 2021;2021:7713058. https://doi.org/10.1155/2021/7713058.
46. Rayyan MR. The use of objective structured clinical examination in dental education- a narrative review. Front Oral Health. 2024;5:1336677. https://doi.org/10.3389/froh.2024.1336677.
47. Cidoncha G, Munoz-Corcuera M, Sanchez V, Pardo Monedero MJ, Antoranz A. The objective structured clinical examination (OSCE) in periodontology with simulated patient: the Most realistic approach to clinical practice in dentistry. Int J Environ Res Public Health. 2023;20(3) https://doi.org/10.3390/ijerph20032661.
48. Park SE, Timothe P, Nalliah R, Karimbux NY, Howell TH. A case completion curriculum for clinical dental education: replacing numerical requirements with patient-based comprehensive care. J Dent Educ. 2011;75(11):1411–6.

49. Bertoli E, Lawson KP, Bishop SS. Dental students' skills assessments: comparisons of daily clinical grades and clinical and laboratory assessments. J Dent Educ. 2018;82(4):417–23. https://doi.org/10.21815/JDE.018.045.
50. Lundegren N, Lindberg P, Gummesson C. Experiences of the use of portfolio in dental education—a qualitative meta-ethnographic literature review. Eur J Dent Educ. 2024;28(2):567–75. https://doi.org/10.1111/eje.12982.
51. Irwin SP, Durning SJ, Dong T. Examining self-efficacy among recent graduates of postgraduate dental education programs. J Dent Educ. 2024; https://doi.org/10.1002/jdd.13742.
52. Liang L, Lin AJ, Ha V, Chutinan S, Ohyama H. Evaluating dental student self-assessment across preclinical anatomy waxing and operative exercises. J Dent Educ. 2024;88(8):1048–54. https://doi.org/10.1002/jdd.13536.
53. Friedlander LT, Meldrum AM, Lyons K. Curriculum development in final year dentistry to enhance competency and professionalism for contemporary general dental practice. Eur J Dent Educ. 2019;23(4):498–506. https://doi.org/10.1111/eje.12458.
54. Kaur D, Negi G, Jain A, Meinia SK, Sidhu TK, Rathore BB. Structured feedback: a teaching and learning tool for the postgraduate medical students in transfusion medicine. Asian J Transfus Sci. 2023;17(1):13–20. https://doi.org/10.4103/ajts.ajts_127_21.
55. Svensater G, Rohlin M. Assessment model blending formative and summative assessments using the SOLO taxonomy. Eur J Dent Educ. 2023;27(1):149–57. https://doi.org/10.1111/eje.12787.
56. McMullen J, Arakawa N, Anderson C, Pattison L, McGrath S. A systematic review of contemporary competency-based education and training for pharmacy practitioners and students. Res Social Adm Pharm. 2023;19(2):192–217. https://doi.org/10.1016/j.sapharm.2022.09.013.
57. Bateman HL, McCracken GI. Patient feedback applied in undergraduate dental education for individual student development and assessment: a scoping review. Eur J Dent Educ. 2024;28(4):1025–35. https://doi.org/10.1111/eje.13037.
58. Nasseripour M, Agouropoulos A, Van Harten MT, Correia M, Sabri N, Rollman A. Current state of professionalism curriculum in oral health education. Eur J Dent Educ. 2025;29(1):92–103. https://doi.org/10.1111/eje.13048.
59. Beckman TJ, Cook DA, Mandrekar JN. What is the validity evidence for assessments of clinical teaching? J Gen Intern Med. 2005;20(12):1159–64. https://doi.org/10.1111/j.1525-1497.2005.0258.x.
60. O'Donnell JA, Oakley M, Haney S, O'Neill PN, Taylor D. Rubrics 101: a primer for rubric development in dental education. J Dent Educ. 2011;75(9):1163–75. https://doi.org/10.1002/j.0022-0337.2011.75.9.tb05160.x.
61. Furze J, Gale JR, Black L, Cochran TM, Jensen GM. Clinical reasoning: development of a grading rubric for student assessment. J Phys Ther Educ. 2015;29(3)
62. Haj-Ali R, Feil P. Rater reliability: short- and long-term effects of calibration training. J Dent Educ. 2006;70(4):428–33. https://doi.org/10.1002/j.0022-0337.2006.70.4.tb04097.x.
63. Nayakar R, Sardesai P, Killedar S, Patil A, Kakodker M. Knowledge, awareness and practices of the use of digital technology in dentistry among postgraduate students and dental practitioners in India: a cross-sectional study. J Clin Diagn Res. 2022;16(2)
64. Kim KJ, Kim G, Kang Y. Faculty perceptions and use of e-learning resources for medical education and future predictions. Korean J Med Educ. 2023;35(4):325–34. https://doi.org/10.3946/kjme.2023.270.
65. Buchanan JA. Use of simulation technology in dental education. J Dent Educ. 2001;65(11):1225–31. https://doi.org/10.1002/j.0022-0337.2001.65.11.tb03481.x.
66. du Plooy E, Casteleijn D, Franzsen D. Personalized adaptive learning in higher education: a scoping review of key characteristics and impact on academic performance and engagement. Heliyon. 2024;10(21):e39630. https://doi.org/10.1016/j.heliyon.2024.e39630.
67. Atkinson JC, Zeller GG, Shah C. Electronic patient records for dental school clinics: more than paperless systems. J Dent Educ. 2002;66(5):634–42. https://doi.org/10.1002/j.0022-0337.2002.66.5.tb03542.x.

68. Eden CA, Chisom ON, Adeniyi IS. Harnessing technology integration in education: strategies for enhancing learning outcomes and equity. World J Adv Eng Technol Sci. 2024;11(2):001–8.
69. Salian A, Sanal Kumar S, Natarajan S, Lewis AJ, Manaktala N, Naik DG, et al. Performance of dental students in understanding and retention of oral pathology concepts: a comparative analysis of traditional versus live-field teaching methods. ScientificWorldJournal. 2022;2022:3257377. https://doi.org/10.1155/2022/3257377.
70. Bin Rubaia'an MA. Dental education: a guide for novice tutors. Cureus. 2023;15(8):e43227. https://doi.org/10.7759/cureus.43227.
71. Nizami MZI, Xue VW, Wong AWY, Yu OY, Yeung C, Chu CH. Challenge-based learning in dental education. Dent J (Basel). 2023;11(1):14. https://doi.org/10.3390/dj11010014.
72. Niemi H. Active learning—a cultural change needed in teacher education and schools. Teach Teach Educ. 2002;18(7):763–80. https://doi.org/10.1016/s0742-051x(02)00042-2.
73. Caldwell D, Sortino M, Winnington J, Cresswell-Yeager TJ. Comprehensive faculty development. In: Kyei-Blankson L, Ntuli E, Blankson J, editors. Handbook of research on creating meaningful experiences in online courses. Advances in educational technologies and instructional design. Hershey: IGI Global; 2020. p. 25–36.
74. Islam NM, Laughter L, Sadid-Zadeh R, Smith C, Dolan TA, Crain G, et al. Adopting artificial intelligence in dental education: a model for academic leadership and innovation. J Dent Educ. 2022;86(11):1545–51. https://doi.org/10.1002/jdd.13010.
75. Zhang Y, Stokes J, Anselmi L, Bower P, Xu J. Can integrated care interventions strengthen primary care and improve outcomes for patients with chronic diseases? A systematic review and meta-analysis. Health Res Policy Syst. 2025;23(1):5. https://doi.org/10.1186/s12961-024-01260-1.
76. Kaushik R, Rapaka R. AI-driven evolution in teledentistry: a comprehensive overview of technology and clinical applications. Dent Rev. 2025;5(2):100154. https://doi.org/10.1016/j.dentre.2025.100154.
77. Pyle MA. New models of dental education and curricular change: their potential impact on dental education. J Dent Educ. 2012;76(1):89–97.
78. Asogwa VC. Global Best practices in education: a conceptual definition and criticisms. J Res Initiat. 2024;8(3):9.
79. Ta A, D'Souza G, Augustine V. Effect of professional development programme on mentorship in enhancing self-efficacy and outcome expectancy of in-service teachers. Int J Educ Reform. 2025;0(0):10567879251323882. https://doi.org/10.1177/10567879251323882.
80. Hobson R, Rolland S, Rotgans J, Schoonheim-Klein M, Best H, Chomyszyn-Gajewska M, et al. Quality assurance, benchmarking, assessment and mutual international recognition of qualifications. Eur J Dent Educ. 2008;12 Suppl 1(s1):92–100. https://doi.org/10.1111/j.1600-0579.2007.00484.x.
81. Lomas L, Nicholls G. Enhancing teaching quality through peer review of teaching. Qual High Educ. 2005;11(2):137–49. https://doi.org/10.1080/13538320500175118.

A Fresh Look at the Good Old Lecture

3

R. M. Baiju

3.1 Introduction

The term lecture is derived from 'legere', a Latin word meaning '*to read*' or '*read aloud*'. The history of lectures can be traced back to the fifth century, which has roots in religious practices of reading aloud holy books like the Bible. Books were rare at that time, and hence books kept on a podium were read aloud for people to listen to. Reading was almost similar to lecturing in the initial days. Ex tempore was an exception, as deviating from the text whilst lecturing was not considered appropriate. The art of lecturing has undergone tremendous transformation over hundreds of years and has attained its current form with the intellectual contribution and public communication skills of the lecturer assuming significant importance. The transformation towards this began as early as the 1970s by Fichte, a German Professor who started lecturing without a text [1].

Lecture may be defined as a structured oral presentation to a large group by an expert in the concerned field with the help of facts, figures and other visual aids. A lecture is still a very important didactic instructional method in education where the teacher acts as the primary information provider [2]. Unless planned intentionally, a lecture may often remain as a one-way communication from the expert teacher who stands and delivers whilst the students remain passive. The transfer of communication in a lecture may happen in many ways, including verbal, extra-verbal, non-verbal and visual. In verbal communication, words convey a message through descriptions, explanation, observations and by giving examples. Extra-verbal communications happens through a skillful way of speaking, through clarity of words, fluency, audibility, pace, intonation and occasional pauses. The majority of communication happens without the usage of words. In non-verbal communication,

R. M. Baiju (✉)
Government Dental College, Kottayam, Kerala, India

Kerala University of Health Sciences, Thrissur, Kerala, India

R. M. Baiju, S. Thomas (eds.), *The Dental Teacher*,
https://doi.org/10.1007/978-3-032-07551-2_3

effective usage of body language is important. Information transfer happens through facial expressions, gestures and body movements, eye contact and positions. The visual element of communication is an integral component in a lecture, which may be enhanced with the use of additional visual aids. The most important visual aid in a lecture is the lecturer himself or herself. Students learn in multiple ways in a lecture. They listen, observe, ask doubts, engage in discussion and take notes.

During the last one and half centuries, dental education has progressed steadfastly by leaps and bounds. Medical and dental education ideally aims to create competent professionals with knowledge, skills and the right attitudes. Although there are different teaching-learning methods available for undergraduate dental education, like most disciplines, didactic sessions or lectures still remain an important component of medical education.

3.2 The Quintessential Lecture Format

Traditional lecture is still one of the major modes of instruction in present-day dental education. One of the salient features of a lecture is the possibility of transmitting the teacher's personal perspective about the lesson being presented. The complex concepts are simplified in a lecture, and students have the opportunity to clarify their doubts. In a lecture, learning happens in multiple ways, including observing, listening, summarising and writing lecture notes. Lectures can provide a good summary of the topic, and a similar summary can be made by the student only through labourious, time-consuming reading. Traditional lecture format needs a reassessment, as there are several inadequacies inherent in it. It is now widely recognised that deep learning occurs with students' involvement and interaction [3]. Online/virtual lectures are a new addition since the pandemic. Time flexibility, especially if the class is recorded, is a huge advantage compared to face-to-face lectures. The ability to stop attending and resuming lectures according to convenience is another benefit. There is a possibility to better understand complex concepts and easy access to shared materials [4].

3.3 Advantages of Lecture as an Instructional Method

- Effective lecturers can influence students by their charisma. As students, we still cherish good lectures that we enjoyed during our student days.
- Transmission of important facts in a straightforward, easy manner directly to students attending the class.
- Ideal for introducing any course or topic, which may be further dealt with by other instructional methods.
- A lecture performance by a skilful teacher with good oratory skills in a theatre-like setting can create a lasting impact about the topic among the students.
- Inspiring lectures help to build good student-teacher relationships that may lead to improved learning outcomes and positive learner behaviour.

- Lectures can be customised based on time, curriculum and audience.
- Good for teaching large groups.
- There are different types of learners. Lectures promote the auditory learners, those learners who like to listen.
- Lecture notes can be ideal learning material, as they may be prepared by the experienced teacher after much reference.
- Highly cost-effective at the same time as reaching a larger audience.

3.4 Disadvantages of Conventional Lecture [5]

- The effectiveness of a lecture depends heavily on the lecturing skills of the teacher.
- Usually non-engaging, where students remain passive.
- Cannot maintain student's attention throughout the duration of the lecture.
- Teachers rarely get feedback regarding the extent and depth of learning that happened.
- One-size-fits-all approach—all students do not learn at the same pace.
- Information got from lecture is not retained if the students do not read further and learn about the lecture topic after the lecture.
- Not ideal for teaching the higher orders of cognitive domain like application, analysis and synthesis.
- Difficult for those learners who have a learning style other than auditory.
- Those who missed the live lecture also missed the experience.
- Often monotonous with information overload.

3.5 Drawbacks of Lecture as an Instructional Method

Drawback include limitations of the lecturer and pedagogical limitations. Personal limitations include language and vocabulary, confidence, depth of understanding of the topic and teaching experience. Such deficits ultimately lead to inferior learning outcomes. Such limitations undermine the self-confidence of the teachers, further leading to negative student feedback. Lectures have innate limitations in pedagogy. The *Bloom's Taxonomy*, the foundational principle in teaching and learning, comprises three domains: the knowledge domain the skills domain and the attitudes domain. Lectures have limitations in providing instructions in skills and attitude domains. All experienced teachers understand its limitations in imparting learning activities with respect to the knowledge domain itself.

Only when a lecture combines the transfer of information and incorporates interactive techniques for active student engagement, does it become a highly effective instructional method [6].

3.6 Interactive Learning Approaches

Several innovations have transformed the traditional lecture to suit the changing needs of the modern-day dental curriculum. Over the last couple of decades, several curricular reforms have suggested the need for effective delivery of information to students through lecture. Promotion of active learning has been suggested as a strategy to enhance teaching efficiency for attainment of improved learning outcomes [7]. Active learning happens when students proactively engage not only with the learning resources but also among themselves to learn together. Interactive lecture sessions can enhance long-term retention of concepts through active learner engagement. Students feel more responsible for their learning. This collaborative or team learning happens through improved interaction among peers as well as through enhanced teacher-student interaction, which could improve the student's presentation skills and confidence.

The Flipped Classroom Is an interactive learning attempt to provide a more customised and personalised education to the learners in a large group setting. The concept was originally mooted by Jonathan Bergman and Aaron Sams, two chemistry teachers, in 2007. The idea of the conventional classroom is flipped so that what is traditionally done at home is done in a flipped classroom and what is usually done in a traditional classroom is now done at the learner's home [8]. Essentially flipped class room is a blended learning strategy that aims to deliver the instructional content outside of the classroom, mostly in an online mode. The kind of content delivered includes online videos, slides, printed literature, website resources, etc. The learning resources are made available to the students well in advance of the class, and clear directions are given on what to be prepared and how it is to be delivered in the forthcoming class. The precious classroom time is spent on the application of the learnt content. The classroom activity may be in the form of problem solving, project-based discussion, quizzes, experiments, presentations by one student or a group of students, or role plays. According to Jon Bergmann, the flipped classroom model enables learning at the higher levels of *Bloom's Taxonomy* like application, analysis, evaluation and creation.

The merits of a flipped classroom include:

- Students get the opportunity to learn content at home at their own pace.
- The teacher can effectively use the class time for interactive discussion and collaboration.
- High possibility for deep learning as students engage with the content more intensely in the class through proctored interaction.
- Benefits both slow learners and advanced learners as they help each other in solving problems during the class.
- Equal learning opportunities—teachers can pay more attention during class to students or groups, especially to those who need more attention in learning.

The limitations include:

- Students need access to technology, which may be an issue with resource-poor settings.
- Effective learning at home can happen only with students' self-discipline.
- Unavailability of a teacher may hinder learning the content at home.

Spaced Learning Methodology Is another less studied interactive instructional model. It involves multiple highly intense learning sessions interspersed with periods of inactivity or leisure. During the breaks distractor activities are implemented [9]. Memory is the encoding, storage and retrieval of information with the functioning of the brain. Essentially there are two kinds of memory: short-term and long-term memory. Messages received by students are initially temporarily stored in short-term memory. Short-term memory can hold a small amount of information for a brief period of time, say a few seconds and it is rapidly forgotten. Incomprehensible facts or difficult-to-understand concepts are not stored. In long-term memory, information is semantically stored for longer periods. Stories are easier to retrieve than conceptual facts when stored in the long-term memory. The information enters working memory prior to it being stored in long-term memory. Visual clues are important in medical and dental education. Procedures and concepts that are conveyed with the help of visual aids are linked to long-term memory. Any instructional method ideally aims at promoting long-term memory. Practice and repetition are methods to enable long-term memory. Clinical conditions taught based on real-life patient stories are often easily retrieved long after because of the peculiarity of the episodic narrative element they have. Spaced learning with repetitive interstitial distractor breaks may result in deep learning and the creation of long-term memory [10]. A study conducted in a Malaysian dental school reported that the flipped classroom model and spaced learning methodology fared superior to traditional lecture concerning knowledge gain when assessed immediately after the pedagogical intervention [3].

There are other ways to make lectures interactive. The lecturer may form a *Buzz group* of three or four students, who together solve a problem or give shape to an idea during the class. The outcome may be presented to the entire class. This can add an activity to the class and can serve as a break in lecturing. Students generally respond to questions after a *Buzz group*, as they gain reassurance about their responses from the discussion.

A short quiz on the previous class or the topic just covered in class can be another activity for student engagement. This can be in the form of multiple-choice questions or rapid-fire. Audio-visual clues can add more variety and make the session more interesting.

3.7 Performing Lecture in the Lecture Theatre

The environment in which the lecture takes place influences the effectiveness of the session. The room should be properly lit and ventilated. The indoor temperature should be comfortable. The speaker should be visible to all the students. There must be space for the teacher to move around during the lecture. The speaker should use the podium only to place the lecture notes or text books. He or she should not hide behind it. It is always advisable for the lecturer to ensure all arrangements are in place. The audiovisual aids and public address system, if available, should be checked for proper functioning. The outside environment should not be noisy or distracting. The seating must be arranged so that all students are comfortable and have a good view of the lecturer (Fig. 3.1).

Rules and regulations of the session, if not already informed, can be provided at the outset.

The opening of the lecture is crucial to its success. The introduction sets the tone. The lecturer should plan to make an interesting and captivating opening—perhaps a story or a joke to grab the students' attention. The story should be related to the lesson being delivered. An interesting clinical history of a case can be presented to draw attention to the condition or treatment that is going to be discussed further in the class. Jokes should be used only if they come naturally to the teacher. Sarcasm or humiliation should be avoided, as should racist, sexual, or gender-insensitive remarks. The introduction aims to capture the attention of all students regarding what is going to be taught that day. The enthusiasm, expressiveness, and dynamism

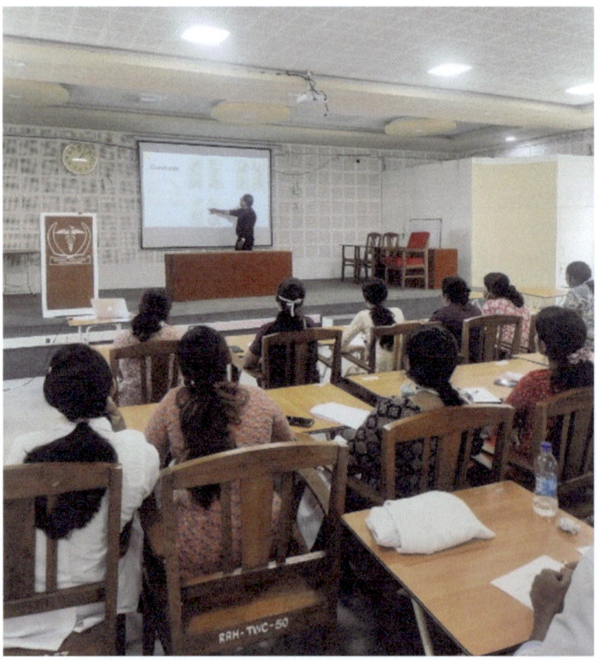

Fig. 3.1 Lecture in progress in a lecture theatre

of the lecturer work wonders among the audience. Examples and analogies related to the topic generate interest and help to sustain it until the end of the class.

Specific learning objectives (SLOs): of the session must be mentioned in the beginning. The statement of objectives should begin as '*At the end of the class, the students will be able to....*'. Ideally, there should be three to five SLOs for one lecture session. More important is the achievement of the set SLOs rather than preparing an over-enthusiastic, extensive list and struggling with it at the end. Be careful to frame the SLOs so that they are specific, measurable, achievable, relevant, and time bound (SMART). Thoughtfully prepared SLOs are critical for the effectiveness of the session. In the context of the competency-based dynamic dental curriculum, the SLOs consist of actionable verbs and reflect an outcome-based approach. At the end of the session, both teachers and students can revisit the SLOs and identify how far the SLOs have been achieved.

The intriguing short introduction is followed by the delivery of the actual lecture content. This is known as the *body* of the lecture. A one- to two-page handout may be given to students based on the content of the class. The handouts can be thoughtfully created as a template with sufficient space between points so that students can use them to write lecture notes.

Throughout the lecture, the movements, gestures and facial expressions of the lecturer hold the key. A good lecturer always keeps moving and makes themselves the most significant visual aid. Maintaining a happy face is better than a gloomy one during teaching. The speaker's gaze should reach every corner of the lecture room making eye contact with as many students as possible. This will keep them engaged and attentive. By doing so, the lecturer receives feedback in return about how well their words are received by the audience.

Voice and Pace: Voice and pace of lecturing are critical. Monotone lecturing is monotonous and boring. The lecturer should modulate the voice to create some drama. An occasional pause just before delivering an important point draws maximum attention. Volume and pitch of speech are equally important. Similarly, the pace of lecturing is crucial. The teaching should not be too fast or too slow. Repetition of certain facts is incredible when used judiciously. According to Bryan Doyle, the lecturer should be an actor to some extent [11]. It is documented that *Theatrics* can enhance learning and increase learner satisfaction [12].

Content: Nothing can minimise the value of content in a lecture. The primary objective of the lecture is to inform, and the quality of content drives attainment of the objective. The contents should do justice to the lecture title and should be appropriate to the target audience. A good teacher does not try to teach everything related to the topic being discussed in the given limited lecture time but rather highlights the relevant things related to the topic in the audience's perspective. A good lecture should trigger the desire to learn more. The most important points or the crux of the content should be introduced early in the first 15–30 min. Studies show that contents presented early in the lecture are well received by the students, as it is conveyed within the average attention span [13, 14].

Planning and organising: The importance of planning and organising the lecture well cannot be overemphasised. A good lecturer arrives early, starts the session on time, transfers the information in a logical order and finishes on time. The transition from one point to the other is seamless and important aspects are duly emphasised. There is respect for the needs of the listener. Time is allotted for discussion and feedback towards the end. This approach engages the listener and induces deep learning. A good lecture is nothing short of a stage performance and any good performance needs planning, preparation and rehearsal (Table 3.1).

The lecture should not end abruptly, however short and sweet the lecture may be. Before closure the audience should be informed about it and they should be expecting it. A good summary of the important points informed should be restated before concluding. This improves learning. The summary should be short and precise. Before concluding, check with the audience whether the objectives stated at the outset were met. Lecturers should bravely face the questions from the students and answer them clearly and unambiguously to the possible extent. If the teacher needs to refer and verify further to answer the query, say so promptly. Smart teachers don't answer the student's question straight away; rather, they ask counter questions so as to extract the answer from the students themselves. This is a highly rated technique, as the students will never forget this interaction and will transfer the information to their long-term memory. The teacher's response to the query should be short and to the point. Do not give another lecture. Answer queries of individual students to the entire class after repeating the question so that everyone would benefit out of it. Unnecessary questions and those not directly related to the topic discussed need not be encouraged in the class. Inform the students to contact the teacher during leisure so that all such doubts can be cleared patiently without disturbing other students' time.

Table 3.1 Lecture skills

Lecturing skills	
Preparation	Consider the audience dynamics Time allotted Learning objectives
Openings	To grab attention Establish rapport Provide lecture structure
Explaining	The core skill Clarity, generating interest and persuasion are critical
Narrating	A powerful skill to instil curiosity Tell a patient's story, incident or personal experience
Comparing and contrasting	Have a clear outline of what is to be compared and how to do it
Audio visual aids	Plan what, when and how to use. Beware to use it judiciously
Responsiveness to audience	Closely observing the audience, monitoring their reactions and responding accordingly
Interactive engagements	Improve attentiveness and enhance learning. Keeps them involved
Summarising	Used in between a lecture and at the end. Should emphasise the key points

Adapted from AMEE Medical Education Guide No. 22: Refreshing lecturing: a guide for lecturers [15]

Table 3.2 The *big five* classroom management strategy [17]

1	Establish classroom rules for expectations regarding student behaviour
2	Build classroom routines for formal disciplined instruction
3	Reinforce positive behaviour using praise and rewards
4	Manage misbehaviour consistently and appropriately
5	Foster student interaction and engagement to promote active learning in class room

Giving handouts is good as part of a lecture for large groups. There are different types of handouts. *Outlines* are a short summary of not more than one page with some key references. *Interactive handouts* are given during the lecture where there is some problem or activity to be done to fill in the blanks. Another type is *key information handouts* containing some special diagrams, formulae, references or quotations. *Full handouts* are the complete text of the lecture. This perhaps will make the students less attentive, as they think that even if they do not pay attention to the lecture, they are safe since they have the handouts. Yet another type is the *tasks and problems handouts,* which basically contain the problems and/or tasks used in the lecture. Interactive handouts are better than full handouts in driving learning and better student engagement [16]. Five different classroom management strategies are listed in Table 3.2.

3.8 Different Lecturing Styles

Every lecturer has his/her own style influenced by observing their teachers, seniors or peers. Brown and Bhakthar, in a rigorous cluster analysis of responses to a set of questions, have identified five distinct lecturing styles [18].

- ***Oral presenters***: They merely read aloud texts in a monotonous manner. No attempt to communicate and engage. No writing on the board or use of the visual aids.
- ***Visual information givers***: They confidently rely on projection software to provide full content of their class. They explain with the help of diagrams or images and explain complex relationships and concepts. They provide the full lecture notes and allow students time to copy whatever is presented.

Table 3.3 Lecturer types

1	Authoritarian	Has good control over the class. Strong emphasis on rules. Strict punishment for inappropriate behaviour. Often intimidating. Not collaborative in learning approach
2	Authoritative	Firm yet fair. Due respect to students. Expect participatory and collaborative approaches from students. Ideal management style for both students and teachers
3	Permissive	Low control, less student engagement for learning, and no rules. Disorderly conduct of the class
4	Indulgent	Students are free to make their own decisions in classroom. Students see them as friends. Unpredictable learning

- ***Exemplary performers***: They confidently perform the lecture through thorough planning and execution. They prepare the content based on answers to certain questions that students would want to know. They organise the lecture under headings, subheadings and explanations. The different lecturer types are presented in Table 3.3.
- ***Eclectic lecturers***: Although they use different techniques, including humour, to enthuse the students, they lack confidence in their lecturing abilities. They often find it difficult to select a topic and to organise the lecture.
- They are often overconfident that they under prepare for their sessions. They are ill organised and the lecture lacks objectives. They dishonour the essential requisites of a lecture.

- Now we can relate ourselves to one of the said lecture styles, partially if not completely.

3.9 Different Lecture Organisational Styles

The following are the different lecture structures identified in literature [5, 18].

- *The classical:* the most common and easiest way of lecture structuring under headings and subheadings like clinical presentation, diagnoses, prognosis and management.
- *The problem centred:* A problem is presented at the outset and the solution to it follows. This style can generate some curiosity among the clinical students.
- *The sequential:* following presentation of a problem, a series of reasoning is provided leading to the solution.
- *The comparative:* this style essentially tries to compare two models or perspectives. A common drawback is that the audience may not be aware of the perspectives being discussed.
- *The thesis:* an assertion is made at the outset. The narration then tries to prove or disprove. This can be an interesting approach for certain students.

- Most lectures are a mixture of the above organisational styles with a little bias of one or the other style. The organisational style, if mentioned to the audience is well received, irrespective of the structure of the lecture.

3.10 Effective Use of Audiovisual Aids

The era of the blackboard has come to an end. Whiteboards and coloured markers have replaced the dusty blackboards. Post pandemic, the current lecturer heavily depends on the PowerPoint presentation. The overuse or abuse of the presentation software is boring and detracts audience attention in a lecture. The long, overextended, repetitive and distracting presentation where the speaker reads every word projected on screen is popularly known as "*death by power point*". Several factors contribute to death by PowerPoint, including too many slides, overly crowded slides, meaning fewer graphics, and the speaker simply reading the slides in a monotone.

- PowerPoint is just an aid, not everything in a lecture.
- Employ the projection appropriately in a lecture.
- Slides should complement the lecture.
- Ideal for showing clinical photos, images or videos for better learning.
- Text colour should contrast the background colour.
- Ideally one idea per slide.
- Follow the 5/5/5 rule-5 lines per slide, five words per line and less than five text heavy slides in a row.
- Use bullet points—short phrases or key words rather than long sentences.
- Employ multimedia in slides to engage different learning styles. Interactive panel is the new gadget in the classroom. with an internet connection, videos can be played and multimedia files can be projected for the benefit of the students.

3.11 Lecture Attendance

There are several factors that contribute to students' attendance in lecture classes. Primarily because of the mandatory attendance required to sit for the examination. Attendance drops for non-mandatory lectures. Undoubtedly significant learning happens in lectures, as one reported higher examination grades for those students who regularly attended lectures [19]. The timing of the lecture is one thing. Generally attendance is less for early morning lectures when compared to other schedules. Similarly, lecture classes on the day just before the beginning of holidays and soon after the end of vacation generally have less attendance irrespective of the teacher or the subject. Factors that help to increase lecture attendance include the ability of a lecturer to communicate with clarity and a lecture that is structured and well organised [20]. Command of the subject comes only next to communication skills, according to student feedback. Personality traits of the lecturer influence student' interest in attending the class [21]. This observation underscores the importance of harnessing professionalism among dental educators.

3.12 Evaluation of Lecture

The primary objective of evaluation is self-assessment of lecturing abilities. The purpose is constructive or developmental—to improve lecturing. The evaluation can be done through students' academic performance or examination scores. But more practically, immediate student feedback, peer assessment and self-evaluation are more direct and beneficial. Students' feedback can be obtained after each session or periodically through physical forms or Google Forms preserving students' anonymity. Rating scales may be provided to facilitate easy responding. There is an observation suggesting that students' feedback should be used with caution [22]. Reflections on practice is another sought after evaluation method. The responses of student feedback and peer feedback are collected and analysed. After careful thought, consideration and a little bit of research, modifications are made and the cycle continues.

Reflections on practice are excellent way for evaluating lecture skills. But it requires effort, insight and an open-mindedness to embrace change.

3.13 Conclusion

Lecture is still the most popular instructional method in dental education. It is highly efficient and economical for large group teaching. Good teachers are not born, but they are created. Any ordinary skilled dentist or dental specialist can become a good lecturer. The teacher has to be willing to learn and self-develop throughout the career. Lifelong learning can be accomplished through faculty refresher courses and integrated self-directed learning. The teacher should be willing to accept criticism and positively respond to student feedback and earnestly make all attempts to improve the lecturing style. Newer innovations, including interactive learning approaches and judicious use of audio-visual aids and technology are making the good old lecture a highly effective teaching learning method even in the present times.

References

1. Chandrasekharan Nair K, et al. Lecture remains to be an effective method of teaching in dental education. Acta Sci Dent Sci. 2022;6(3):10.
2. Billings-Gagliardi S, Mazor KM. Students' decision about lecture attendance: do electronic course matter? Acad Med. 2007;82(10 Suppl):S73–6.
3. Kohli S, Sukumar AK, Zhen CT, Yew AS, Gomez AA. Dental education: lecture versus flipped and spaced learning. Dent Res J. 2019;16:289–97.

4. Bartok-Nicolae C, Raftu G, Briceag R, Sachelarie L, Caraiane A, Duta M, Farcas DM. Virtual and traditional lecturing technique impact on dental education. Appl Sci. 2022;12:1678. https://doi.org/10.3390/app12031678.
5. Bligh DA. Whats the use of lectures? New York: Jossey Bass; 2000.
6. Cardall S, Krupat E, Ulrich M. Live lecture versus video- recorded lecture: are students voting with their feet? Acad Med. 2008;83:1174–8.
7. Shrivastava RB, Lal S, Shrivastava SP. Is it time to say goodbye or introduce specific strategies to enhance their effectiveness. Curr Med Issues. 2022;20(4):259–61.
8. Bergmann J, Sams A. Flip your class room: reach every student in every class every day. Eugene: International Society for Technology in Education; 2012.
9. Kelley P, Whatson T. Making long-term memories in minutes: a spaced learning pattern from memory research in education. Front Hum Neurosci. 2013;7:589.
10. Sweller J, van Merriënboer JJ, Paas FG. Cognitive architecture and instructional design. Educ Psychol Rev. 1998;10:251–96.
11. Doyle BB. Medical lecturing as good theater. Presented at the Seminar on Medical Education. Bethesda: UNformed Services Medical School; 1986.
12. Naftulin DH, Ware JE Jr, Donnelly FA. The doctor fox lecture: a paradigm of educational seduction. J Med Ed. 1973;48:631–5.
13. Golden AS. Lecure skills in medical education. Indian J Pediatr. 1989;56:29–34.
14. Giles RM, Johnson MR, Knight KE, Zammett S, Weinman J. Recall of lecture information, a question of what, when and where. Med Educ. 1982;16:264–8.
15. Brown G, Manogue M. AMEE Medical Education Guide No. 22: refreshing lecturing: a guide for lecturers. Med Teach. 2001;23(3):231–44. https://doi.org/10.1080/01421590120043000. PMID: 12098394
16. Hartley J. Designing instructional text. 4th ed. London: Kogan Page; 1994.
17. Greenberg J, Putman H, Walsh K. Training our future teachers: class room management. National Council on Teacher Quality; 2014. www.nctq.org/teacherprep
18. Brown GA, Bakhtar M. Styles of lecturing: a study and its implications. Res Pap Educ. 1987;3:131–53.
19. Dhaliwal U. Absenteeism and under achievement in final year medical students. Nat Med J India. 2003;16(1):34–7.
20. Massingham P, Herrington T. Does attendance matter? An examination of students' attitudes, participation, performance and attendance? J Univ Teach Learn Pract. 2006;3(2):83–103.
21. Bollemier SG, Wenger PJ, Fornaish AB. Impact of online lecture-capture on student outcomes in a therapeutic course. Am J Pharm Educ. 2010;74(7):1–5.
22. Ramsden P. Learning to teach in higher education. London: Routledge; 1992.

Teaching Dentistry in Small Groups

4

Biju Thomas

4.1 Introduction

Professional dental education in the various dental schools across the globe happens in classrooms, clinical settings and outreach dental rural centres. The theoretical aspects are taught at the institution/university level and the clinical training is provided at the various specialty and general dentistry clinics in the institution.

Evidence available suggests that small group teaching can provide a more effective platform to improve student learning in medical professional education and the same can be applicable to dental professional education also [1].

A student's ability to effectively understand a topic is increased when they are in an environment wherein they are able to compare their knowledge with other students under the guidance of their peers [2, 3].

Small group teaching thus provides the students an opportunity to work closely with their colleagues which will promote team-building skills which will be useful in their carriers ahead.

Fisher and Ellis [4] reported that the sharing element among members is the key factor which defines the existence of the group. The sharing can be based around perceptions, goals, tasks, etc. Group dynamics greatly influence the sharing pattern. Another defining element is the structure of the group, including the roles, norms, values and power relationships, which can play an important role in the success of interaction in a group because small group teaching also requires maximum interaction among its members, helping them to clarify their understanding and contribute to one another's learning.

A small group teaching programme does not merely mean a small number but refers to the way the teacher works with the group to facilitate the learning process.

B. Thomas (✉)
Department of Periodomtology, AB Shetty Memorial Institute of Dental Sciences, Nitte University, Mangalore, India
e-mail: bijunicy@yahoo.ac.uk

R. M. Baiju, S. Thomas (eds.), *The Dental Teacher*,
https://doi.org/10.1007/978-3-032-07551-2_4

A small group can consist of anywhere between 6 and 12 students with a teacher, but in a dental clinical scenario, it can be as few as two to three students. Conversely, small groups can also be as large as 20–30 students.

It has to be understood in this context that small group learning will be helpful only if the students involve themselves actively in the programme [5]. Studies reported also show that, for long-term retention, the ability to apply the knowledge acquired, critical thinking and the development of a positive attitude, small group classes are better [6, 7].

The main advantage of small group teaching is that it provides an avenue for learning which cannot be obtained in a large group, but the flip side is that it can be more difficult to organise because of the need for more resources such as more additional teachers, space and increased time requirements.

Small group learning should have three active components: active participation by all members, face-to-face contact between the participants and various purposeful activities [8].

If successfully implemented with all three components involved, it can enhance the students' learning experience in several ways, such as addressing gaps in knowledge, developing skills in critical thinking and problem solving, and fostering leadership skills. It also gives students an opportunity to share their ideas and give and receive feedback.

4.2 Role of the Facilitator

The teacher as a facilitator of learning has to manage the group and its activities by asking open-ended questions, guiding the thought process and task, enabling the students to actively participate and express their ideas.

Richmond (1984) has listed five key roles of the teacher, where all he is required to do is to intervene to maintain the group as a cohesive functional unit [9].

(a) To start and finish the group work—maintain time, ensure outcomes are achieved and the tasks clearly explained and the learning needs are met when the activities are finished.
(b) Ensure that the flow of content is maintained—learning should follow in a logical sequence.
(c) Manage the group dynamics.
(d) Facilitate achievement of goals—of the current session and also the overall curriculum, especially those identified by the learners themselves.
(e) Manage the physical and psychological environment of the group.

Tuckman explained a model of group process to describe how group dynamics develop over time [10].

1. Forming—the initial formation of the group. It is the duty of the facilitator to brief the various group members about the activities and purposes of the groups.

He should also introduce all the members and put the participants at ease. To advance from here to the next stage, each member must relinquish the comfort zone of non-threatening topics and risk the possibility of conflict.
2. Norming—in norming, the general guidelines for the group are developed and an exchange of ideas is encouraged within the group. All members are encouraged to be actively involved in the deliberations. The major task function of this stage 3 is the exchange of ideas between group members: They share feelings and ideas and solicit and give feedback to one another. Creativity is high in this stage. Collaboration emerges during this stage when team work ethic and shared leadership are understood by all members.
3. Storming—the group performs the allotted task. If any difference of opinion arises, the moderator assists to solve it. In order to progress to the next stage, group members must move from a 'testing and proving' mentality to a problem-solving mentality. The team members must be able to listen to their teammates and comprehend what they are saying?
4. Performing—the group starts to have a more focused team approach in performing the tasks allotted to it. The performing stage is not reached by all groups. If a group is able to evolve to stage 4, their capacity, range, and depth of personal relations expand to true interdependence. In this stage, people can work independently, in subgroups, or as a total unit with equal competencies.
5. Closure—is the final stage when the group has worked together, finished the tasks allotted and then disbanded. A planned conclusion should include recognition for participation and any achievements and an opportunity for all in the group to say goodbye to each other.

Tuckman's model explains that as the team develops maturity and ability, relationships are established and changes in the style of leadership occur to a more collaborative or shared leadership.

In small group teaching, teams are often forming and changing, and each time that happens, they can move to a different Tuckman stage. A group might be in the Norming or Performing stage, but the addition of a new member might pull them back into the Storming stage, or a team member may miss a meeting, causing the team to fall back into the storming stage. To manage this situation the facilitator should be ready at hand to help the team get back to the performing stage as fast as possible.

4.3 Types of Sessions

The different types of small group sessions in the dental scenario can include case presentations, small group seminars, problem-based learning groups, tutorials, workshops, and so on. When planning the session, keep in mind the resources available, such as infrastructure, equipment, patients, facilitators, and so forth, which are required to achieve the expected learning outcomes.

(a) Seminars: The group discusses the journal article and related content.
(b) Tutorials: students in small groups discuss their essays or doubts on any topic.
(c) Problem classes: To be conducted specifically on topics identified by the group of students as difficult.
(d) Workshops: The facilitator provides input to the group as a whole and also to individual students in the group. The group then works together on the task given.
(e) Problem-based learning: A clinical or theoretical scenario is provided to a group of students who are required to diagnose the problem and provide a solution. The group is expected to meet multiple times to debate the problem, with each student contributing information on the situation and finally arriving at a consensus.

Problem-based learning (PBL) is essentially a student-centred approach in which students master a particular topic or solve a question or problem by working in small groups. The teacher basically functions as an active guide for their students.

The seven broad steps of the PBL process can be stated as:

- Identifying and clarifying the meaning of the question or problem.
- Defining the question or problem.
- Brainstorming and in-depth discussion.
- Restructuring of the question or problem if required.
- Formulation of the learning objectives or goals for the question or problem.
- Independent study.
- Regrouping and synthesis.

Thus, small group teaching can be based on:

(a) Topics such as pulpitis, gingivitis, dental pain, abscesses, and so on.
(b) Clinical case scenarios—where a patient with relevant findings is available or based on case notes.
(c) Situations such as a patient with maxillofacial trauma presenting after a road traffic accident.
(d) Community based-problems affecting sections of the population, such as fluorosis.
(e) Tasks assigned to the learners, such as examination of the soft tissues in the oral cavity or radiographic assessment of the clinical condition in periodontitis and so forth.

The Centre for Teaching Excellence, University of Waterloo, has suggested different types of small group activities as part of group work in the class room [11].

(a) Buzz Groups—can be conducted for any class size with a time frame of 3–10 min. This is a very flexible teaching method where initially the students involve in short informal discussions on a particular question. Then, at a specific moment, the students turn to their adjacent neighbours to discuss any difficulties in understanding the question. The aim is to generate answers or ideas to a particular question, reignite students' interest in the topic and gauge students' understanding.

(b) Think-pair-share—can be done for any class size with a time limit of up to 10 min. This helps to generate ideas, increase students' confidence and improve their participation in larger sessions. The students first answer a question individually and then they are paired and discuss and combine their responses into a joint response, which is then presented to the entire class.

(c) Circle of voices—any class size with a time limit of 10–20 min is suitable. Here, students form groups of four to five. They are given a topic to discuss, and then each student speaks on it for a fixed time limit. This helps generate ideas, improve listening skills, ensure all students participate and create an equal learning environment for everyone.

(d) Rotating trios—it is preferable to have a class size of around 15–30 with a time frame of around10 min. Students discuss issues with many of their classmates by forming trios. A number is allotted to each one in the trio, and then the numbers are rotated among the different trios. This helps students familiarise themselves with their peers, which can be beneficial for generating ideas.

(e) Snowball groups/pyramids—a class size of 15–50 and a time limit of 15–20 min is preferable. Here, students work in doubling groups, first alone, then in pairs, then in fours, and so on. Later, their views are pooled, and one student from each group presents the group's conclusion. This helps develop decision making skills and generate well-vetted ideas.

(f) Jigsaw—can be performed with a class size of between 10 and 50, with a time limit of more than 20 min. The students learn one topic in detail then share their expertise with others. The groups are shuffled so that the students share their knowledge with different group members. This helps deepen understanding of concepts and develop teamwork skills.

(g) Fishbowl—requires a class size of 10–50 and a time of more than 15 min. In this method, one group observes another. The first group forms a circle, and the second group observes the first. Movable seating and ample space are required to implement this. It allows participants to observe group interactions and provides an opportunity for analysis.

(h) Learning teams—can be done with any class and at any time frame. Students are divided into groups of four at the beginning of the term, and all group discussions are carried out within the same learning group. This enables students to get to know their group partners well over the course of the term. This helps to improve interpersonal relationships and boosts confidence for participation in team activities.

The American Board for small group strategies and individual instruction has also recommended various teaching techniques for use with small groups, such as:

(a) Flexible Grouping—students are grouped based on their achievement levels. The basic curriculum is covered for both, but one group may be taught beyond the minimum requirements.
(b) Nominal Brainstorming—each person in the group gets a chance to answer in turn. This cycle continues until all the responses are recorded.
(c) Think-Pair-Share.

Example of a structured dental small group teaching session on periodontal abscess	
Class room teaching	Dental clinical teaching
Desirable outcomes	
Session is planned for fourth BDS students. By the end of the session the student must be able to: Define a periodontal abscess. Identify the signs of an abscess. List the symptoms of an abscess. Enumerate the possible etiologies for the abscess. Describe the pathogenesis of abscess formation.	Session is planned for fourth BDS students. By the end of the session the student must be able to: Recognise the classical clinical presentations of an abscess Differentiate a periodontal abscess from a peri apical abscess Be able to understand the overall management of an abscess
Activity	
Class room teaching	Dental clinical teaching
Case based learning format (group of 8–10 students Reading material (text book reference) will be provided Records of a clinical case of periodontal abscess will be provided for students to record history and for investigations The group of students has to work together and make a diagnostic decision based on history and clinical investigation Create a comprehensive treatment plan	Clinical dental chairside format to be used (5–6 students) Students will take a history from the patient and clinically examine the abscess Lack of an ideal case may limit the students' diagnosis and treatment plan Students should establish a rapport with the patients to get their full co-operation for the clinical examination If a patient is non-cooperative then do not procced with the clinical examination
Summary	
As periodontal abscess is a common occurrence in patients with periodontitis, the students should have sufficient understanding of this important condition	Periodontal abscess is a common clinical presentation in periodontitis patients, hence students must be trained for recognise the condition and its management

4.4 Strategies of a Facilitator

Although small group teaching is learner-focused, the role of the facilitator is not passive. The facilitator must initiate the programme by creating an appropriate environment, putting the learners at ease [12]. Ensure a comfortable seating arrangement for the learners, give an introduction to the programme and ensure activities such as games, role plays, drawing competitions etc., are conducted by the groups to enhance interaction. Outline the expectations of the programme and the rules to be followed. Ask questions; observe their performance and understanding of the knowledge and skills to be acquired.

4.5 Importance of Questioning in Small Group Teaching

Asking questions repeatedly in a small group teaching scenario facilitates a learner-centred approach to the learning process. The facilitator will be able to comprehend the learning needs of each student [13]. This will help to improve their responses and interactions. Questioning will promote clinical reasoning, encourage introspection by the learner and also help the facilitator to track the learner's progress. The different types of questioning strategies will elicit different responses, encourage wider thinking and stimulate discussion.

Questioning can be based on clarification of the problem, evidence available to support the clarification, explanation of the clarification, linking it to available data and a conclusion. If any uncertainty is present, it should be stated for further follow-up. Generally, questions asked can be of three types:

(a) Basic questions requiring an answer of yes or no.
(b) Closed questions which have a specific answer and help to ascertain the knowledge of the learner.
(c) Open questions which will arouse curiosity and stimulate critical thinking in the learner; they will also require the learner to have a good understanding of the topic [14].

4.6 Reflection and Feedback

Reflection involves assessing the effectiveness of the facilitation strategies and the attainment of the lesson goals. It is important to comprehensively evaluate the lesson plan for its full coverage and identity potential areas for improvement [15].

Gathering feedback is also vital to support self-reflective practices [15]. Feedback can be collected verbally or in writing. The key take-away points from the session and the areas that require further clarification can be documented. Feedback can also be subjected to validation by peers.

Once feedback has been received:

(a) Analyse it with an open mind.
(b) Avoid dismissing feedback that does not align with the self-reflective process.
(c) Initiate constructive discussion with learners and ask for specific examples related to the feedback provided.

Table 4.1 Salient features of small group teaching

Small group teaching can be carried out in a variety of settings.
Make sure that the facilities are in place for the type of activity to be conducted.
Make sure that the activity remains learner-centred with a variety of activities and active participation by the members.
Use more of open-ended questions to stimulate learners' thinking and assess their progress.
Take feedback and analyse it for possible future improvements.

4.7 Management of Difficult Situations in Small Group Teaching

The salient features of small group teaching are given in Table 4.1. The teacher should be prepared to handle the common issues that comes with academically engaging a small group of students. Some of the common problems associated with managing small groups has been highlighted by Jacques D in 2003 [16].

(a) Teachers lecturing to the learners instead of facilitating a discussion.
(b) Students not engaging in discussion with each other but only answering the facilitator's questions.
(c) Learners not coming prepared for the session.
(d) One student dominating over others and impeding healthy discussion.
(e) Students not inclined to discuss problems but wanting tailor-made solutions to be given to them.

One of the ways to handle these problems is to let the group manage its own issues without interfering, which is possible only if the group is going to remain together in the long run. *The tutor has to intervene to keep the group focused if the group is relatively new or the deadline to perform the task is short* [17–19].

Dominant students: These students summarise the points and can divert the discussion. One way of managing them is to give each one in the group specific tasks with a definite time frame so that the dominant person cannot monopolise the situation.

Quiet learners: Give them time to respond and divide the group into pairs for a specific task, highlighting positively their contributions in the group.

Learners with negative attitude: This type of attitude can affect the others in the group. Hence, encourage these learners to think of positive situations and discourage lengthy debates.

Students who come unprepared for small group activities: Make sure that each learner is accountable to other team members. Start the class by conducting a small test, which will ensure that they come prepared.

Too much of attention focused on the facilitator: the facilitator should limit his contribution to the students' responses by sharing an appropriate clinical experience that will highlight the relevance of the topic.

4.8 Conclusion

Small group teaching techniques can be used in a variety of dental settings, from the dental clinics to pre-clinical setups, medical and surgical wards, as well as class room settings. It helps to stimulate a learner's interest in a topic and increases inter action with other learners. The teacher or facilitator has an important role in ensuring that the group works in coordination and harmony and that all members take part actively in the entire programme.

References

1. Ozgonul L, Alimoglu MK. Comparison of lecture and team based learning in medical ethics education. Nurs Ethics. 2019;26(3):903–13.
2. Lopping KJ. The effectiveness of peer tutoring in further and higher education: a typology and review of literature. High Educ. 1996;32(3):321–45.
3. Burgess A, McGregor D. Peer teacher training for health professional students: a systematic review of formal programs. BMC Med Educ. 2018;18:263. https://doi.org/10.1186/s12909-018-1356-2.
4. Fisher BA, Ellis DG. Small group decision making: communication and the group process. 3rd ed. New York: Mc Graw Hill Publishing Co; 1990.
5. Kitchen M. Facilitating small groups : how to encourage student learning. Clin Teach. 2012;9(1):3–8.
6. Kleinsasser RC, McKeachie WJ. Teaching tips: strategies , research and theory for college and university teachers. Mod Lang J. 2011;78(4):545.
7. Jacques D. Small group teaching. Oxford Centre for Staff and Learning Development; 2004.
8. Newble D, Cannon R. A handbook for medical teachers. 4th ed. Dordrecht: Kluwer Academic Publishers; 2001.
9. Richmond DE. Improving the effectiveness of small group learning with stratregic intervention. Med Teach. 1984;6(4):138–41.
10. Tuckman BW. Developmental sequence in small groups. Psycol Bull. 1965;63:384–99.
11. (2024) Group work in the classroom: types of small groups. Centre for Teaching Excellence, University of Waterloo.
12. van Diggele C, Burgess A, Mellis C. Planning, preparing and structuring a small group teaching session. BMC Med Educ. 2020;20:462.
13. Mckimm J, Morris C. Small group teaching. Br J Hosp Med (Lond). 2009;70(11):654–7.
14. Watts M, Pedrusa H. Cause and effect of asking questions: reflective case studies from undergraduate sciences. Can J Sci Math Technol Educ. 2005;5:437–52.
15. Lake TR, Vikrey AW, Ryan G. Teaching on the run tips7: effective use of questions. Med J Aust. 2005;182(3):126–7.
16. Jacques D. Teaching small group. In: Cantillon P, Huchinson L, Wood D, editors. IBMJ ABC of learning and teaching Medicine. London: BMJ Publishing Group. p. 19–21.
17. Kitchen M. Facilitating small groups: how to encourage student learning. Clin Teach. 2012;9(1):3–8. https://doi.org/10.1111/j.1743-498X.2011.00493.x. PMID: 22225884
18. McKimm J, Morris C. Small group teaching. Br J Hosp Med (Lond). 2009;70(11):654–7. https://doi.org/10.12968/hmed.2009.70.11.45059. PMID: 20081595
19. Edmunds S, Brown G. Effective small group learning: AMEE guide no. 48. Med Teach. 2010;32(9):715–26. https://doi.org/10.3109/0142159X.2010.505454. PMID: 20795801

Self-Directed Learning: Fundamental Principles

5

Adejumoke A. Adeyemi and Claire Newey

5.1 Learning Outcomes

By the end of this chapter, the dental teacher should be able to:

- Describe what self-directed learning is and understand its relevance to dental education.
- Be aware of the models of self-directed learning and their key features.
- Be able to describe the reflection cycle and identify a model of self-reflection.
- Be aware of how to identify the stage of self-directed learning (SDL) of their students.
- To understand how to set meaningful goals.
- Identify support strategies that help learners to gain skills needed to become successful self-directed learners.
- Be aware of coaching and how this can support the acquisition of self-directedness.
- Be aware of the role of an academic advisor and the evidence base supporting this approach.
- Be aware of peer-assisted learning and peer support.

5.2 Introduction

Dental professionals require the ability to update and develop their skills and knowledge throughout their practising careers so that their clinical skills and knowledge remain up to date in the ever-changing landscape of dentistry. To do this, clinicians

A. A. Adeyemi (✉) · C. Newey
School of Dentistry, Institute of Life Course and Medical Sciences, University of Liverpool, Liverpool, UK
e-mail: aadeyemi@liverpool.ac.uk; cnewey@liverpool.ac.uk

R. M. Baiju, S. Thomas (eds.), *The Dental Teacher*,
https://doi.org/10.1007/978-3-032-07551-2_5

must be able to identify gaps in their knowledge and seek out learning opportunities which will address these areas. The process where individuals take responsibility for identifying what they want to learn is known as 'self-directed learning' (SDL).

It is important that dental students are equipped with skills which allow them to continue to develop long after their undergraduate training ends. Many regulators or advisory bodies, such as the General Dental Council in the United Kingdom and the American Dental Association, for example, stipulate the importance of dental professionals maintaining their knowledge and skills throughout their career [1, 2].

This chapter will introduce the concept of 'self-directed learning' and will describe some of the models used to explain this learning style. Dental teachers will be provided with examples of how they can support their students in acquiring the individual skills needed to become self-directed learners.

The concept of self-directed learning was initially described in the 1960s and 1970s [3–5]. Self-directedness challenges traditional methods of learning and teaching and is a process where the learner works to take control of their own learning, where a student may identify their own learning needs, set relevant goals and assess their own progress towards meeting these. This process may occur in a traditional learning environment, but it is also a skill which can be adopted outside of formal education settings [6, 7].

There are several models of self-directed learning. Despite some structural differences, these models each identify a similar set of key personal characteristics and skills which support successful SDL [5–8]. One such example, the Garrison model of self-directed learning, is shown in Fig. 5.1 [8].

Learners require *insight* into their academic progress so that they can identify specific learning needs and set relevant goals. They must then be *motivated* to undertake independent learning and be able to utilise appropriate learning strategies. They must also believe that they have the capability to complete this work and be able to manage their own behaviours to achieve this. This may involve seeking out additional learning opportunities. Students should be able to

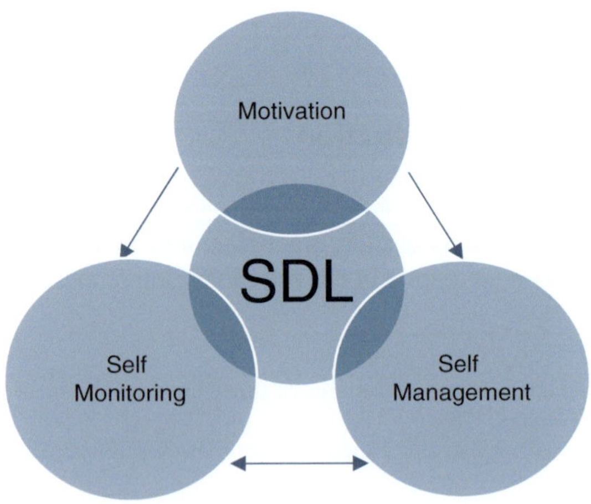

Fig. 5.1 Garrisons model of self-directed learning (SDL) [8]

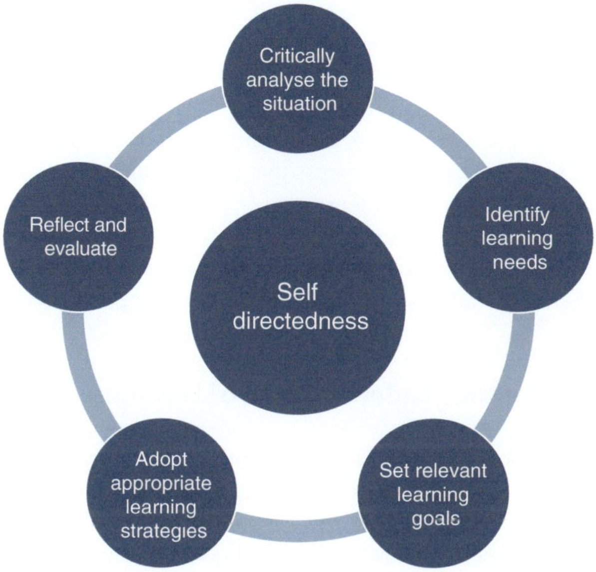
Critically
analyse the
situation
Identify
learning
needs
Set relevant
learning
goals
Adopt
appropriate
learning
strategies
Reflect and
evaluate
Self
directedness

Fig. 5.2 Hammond and Collins' stages to self-directedness [6]

Table 5.1 Attributes for success in self-directed learning (Gavriel 2015)

Attributes for successful self-directedness
Motivation
Self-management
Being able to teach yourself (autodidaxy)
Seek out developmental learning opportunities
Self-reflection and self-assessment

self-monitor their progress. Self-directedness is a cyclical process as reflection and evaluation may lead students to identify further learning goals (Fig. 5.2). The personal attributes that are required to be able to undertake self-directed learning are summarised in Table 5.1.

5.3 Strategies to Support Self-Directed Learning

Dental teachers can have a significant impact in helping students to acquire the skills that are required for self-directed learning (these skills are summarised in Table 5.1 and Fig. 5.2). This section will explore some of the techniques that dental teachers can adopt in their teaching environment to scaffold student development of these skills.

Learning objectives are a useful 'check list' which students can use to compare their current knowledge against to identify areas where they may need to do additional work. Most curricula will have published milestones. Providing students with learning objectives at the start of more formal or didactic teaching such as lectures is commonplace. However, even in informal teaching environments, it can be helpful to briefly describe what students can expect to learn from the session.

Problem based learning (PBL) is now used across multiple disciplines around the world [9–11]. Groups of learners work to identify their own learning objectives and solve problems. This is a learning process that aligns with constructivism, transformational learning and experiential learning [7]. PBL is a student-centred approach where they are encouraged to identify gaps in their knowledge and then go to study and critically evaluate the quality of the learning resources. There are many elements of PBL that help students to foster a self-directed approach to learning [7, 12].

5.3.1 Identifying the Students' Stage of Learning

Self-directedness is not an innate skill. The attributes required to be successful in self-directed learning are skills that can be learned and therefore dental teachers have an important role in helping students acquire these.

The Staged Self-Directed Learning (SSDL) model is a useful tool to help dental teachers identify how mature the learning approach is of the population of students they are teaching [13]. This can provide insight into how much support an individual learner or a group of students may need, and teachers can scaffold strategies to help students advance their learning stage. Grow (1991) proposed that there are four stages associated with adult lifelong learning which, each correlate with a complementary teaching style [13]. The style of tuition the student receives depends on how developed their skills in self-directedness are at that point (Fig. 5.3). Learners may be dependent, interested, involved or self-directed. The teacher can act as an authority figure, a motivator, a facilitator, or a consultant, dependent on the requirements of the students they are teaching. The *dependent* learner relies heavily on instruction from a teacher; at this stage there is no self-direction in their learning. The student can complete tasks set by the teacher but is completely reliant on

x

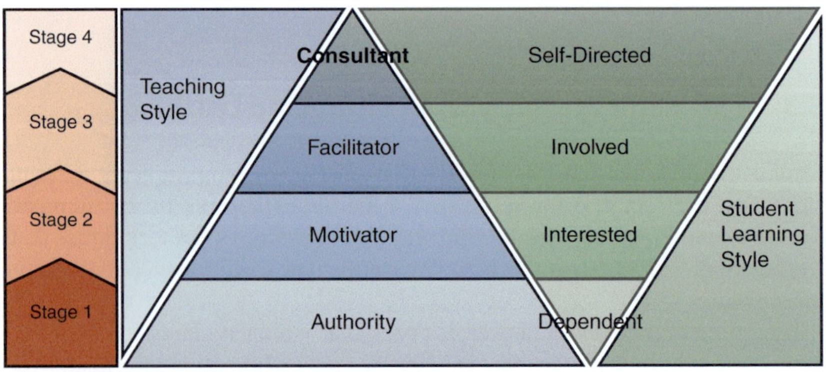

Fig. 5.3 The stages associated with the staged self-directed learning model. (Adapted from [15]

guidance from the teacher, who has an authoritarian role. The *interested* learner can seek out some opportunity to learn and may be able to set personal learning goals but is likely to need support to identify ways to achieve their learning outcomes. They require motivation from the teacher to keep them on track. The *involved* learner is on the way to becoming self-directed; they are beginning to identify some methods to meet their learning goals, and the teacher moves to a facilitating or guiding role. The *self-directed* learner can set their own learning goals and can identify ways to measure success. Their teacher moves into a background position to offer support or consultation (Fig. 5.3).

It is important for dental teachers to consider the stage of training of the students you are working with. The learning stage will impact what skills it would be reasonable for them to currently have and what they are working towards. You may need to adapt your teaching style accordingly. Undergraduate learners early on in their degree programmes will be more likely to be 'dependent' or 'interested' learners than final-year undergraduate students or postgraduate students who may already be working in a self-directed way. It is unwise to opt straight for the 'consultant' approach in an attempt to speed up learner development. It is better to slowly encourage students to progress through each stage of learning until they are ready to have the learning role delegated to them [7, 13].

5.3.2 The What? So What? Now What? Model of Critical Reflection

The What? So What? Now What? The reflective model is commonly used in clinical settings and encourages learners to use three simple questions: 'What?', 'So What?' and 'Now What?' to reflect upon a learning encounter [14]. Learners use guidance questions to direct their thoughts and reflection. This model can be used as a scaffold to help students identify a learning event and analyse the processes and outcomes. It can also help students build their self-management skills by considering how their thoughts and feelings can impact their behaviours and outcomes.

Students are asked to identify an event to reflect upon and then work through the What?, So What? and Now What? stages using the tasks and suggested questions in Table 5.2. The 'What?' stage is intended to be an observational, descriptive, and retrospective process to describe what happened. Enough context should be provided for the scenario to make sense to other readers. When considering, 'So What?' the learner can analyse what could have caused the outcomes, consider their feelings around the event and identify any factors that may be influencing their interpretation of the outcome. This can increase self-awareness of the student and help them to understand the impact they can have on their learning. Finally, in "Now What?" the learner can identify future learning goals and strategies that would help them achieve a desirable outcome. An example of how an undergraduate dental student may use this model is shown in Table 5.3.

Table 5.2 The stages of the 'What? So What? and Now What?' reflective cycle and example questions to consider at each stage

Stage	Task	Suggested questions
What?	Describe the event	What happened? What was the context? Who else was involved? Did anything go well or not well? What did you observe?
So What?	Analyse what happened	Why do you think this happened? How did you feel when it happened? How did these feelings support or hinder you during the experience? What impacts your view of this event? Did you learn any new information? Has this happened before?
Now What?	Identify the next steps	What lessons can you learn from this event? What would you do again in a similar situation? What would you do differently? How can you prepare for a similar situation?

Adapted from [14]

Table 5.3 An example of how a student may utilise the What? So What? Now What? framework during self-reflection

What?	I was using the dental simulator to practise a crown preparation on an upper first molar. This was the first time I had done a molar crown preparation. When I was doing the distal proximal reduction, I created a large undercut on the distopalatal. I did not spot the undercut myself and only became aware of it when my tutor showed it to me. After some work, I did manage to correct the undercut, but it made the tooth preparation over-tapered in this area
So What?	I am still learning and know that I will make mistakes on my first go. I now understand that this is a difficult part of the crown preparation, and I need to take my time. I am pleased that I was able to remove the undercut. When I think about how I created the undercut, I think I blended the proximal reduction into the palatal reduction in one movement and tilted the bur incorrectly going around the "corner" of the tooth
Now What?	I need to practise checking for undercut in the way that my tutor showed me. I will make sure that I am using indirect vision enough. I tried to look directly at the tooth which I think made it harder, and it's also not good for my posture. Next time I am going to complete the proximal and palatal reductions separately and be very careful when I blend the two to make sure my bur is always oriented in the long axis

5.4 Goal Setting

Identifying and setting appropriate goals is a critical element of self-directed learning. Appropriate goals help drive the learning process by providing targets students can work towards. A goal-setting template is a simple tool that can help students to come up with realistic goals that will drive learning forward rather than hinder it. Table 5.4 outlines functions of goals-setting.

SMART goals were outlined by Doran (1984) for use in the business sectors [16]. This goal setting acronym is now commonly used in many workplaces and

Table 5.4 The functions of goals (Locke and Latham 2002) [15]

Functions of goal setting	
Directional	Focus on a particular area
Energising	Increase the level of effort
Increase stamina	Length of time and effort sent
Knowledge	Either gaining new knowledge or consolidating knowledge

Table 5.5 SMARTER goals, adapted from [16]

S	Specific	What is the aim?
M	Measurable	What data will be best used to determine if the goal has been met?
A	Achievable	Is this a realistic goal? Are there appropriate skills and resources available to help you meet it? Is this a goal where you have power over the outcome?
R	Relevant	Does the goal align with the learning needs?
T	Time bound	When is the deadline to accomplish the goal?
E	Evaluated	Has the goal been achieved? If not, are there further goals that can be identified?
R	Reviewed	What have you learned that will further aid your development?

learning environments. To include the evaluative and reflective elements required for self-directed learning, a modified version of this goal setting template, SMARTER, is outlined in Table 5.5.

Students can use the SMARTER goal acronym to help structure their goals. Goal-setting templates, such as shown in Fig. 5.4, can also include sections to support the development of reflection skills. This template exemplar in Fig. 5.4 is adapted from the authors' own institution. It incorporates elements of SMARTER and the What? So What? Now What? approaches, and has been completed from the perspective of a student to illustrate how it may be used in a teaching setting.

5.4.1 Coaching

Coaching, like mentoring, is a strategy aimed at maximising their academic performance. In contrast to mentoring, coaching is a dynamic partnership between coach and student, where the coach works *with* the student to identify ways for the student to achieve their learning goals. To be an effective coach, the dental teacher does not need to have subject knowledge expertise and so all members of the teaching team can have a valuable role in coaching. The key benefits of coaching are outlined in Table 5.6.

Coaching is a dialogue between the dental teacher and the student. One effective way to structure a coaching conversation is to use the GROW model (Table 5.7), which uses a cycle consisting of four stages [17].

These stages do need to be address in this order; however, you may find that for the conversation with the student to flow more naturally, you prefer not to follow the order of the acronym.

Goal Setting Template
What type of goal is this?
An academic goal
Where is this reflection from?
My exam results
What?
Describe what you experienced, what your thoughts were, or what happened that led you to identify this goal. My exam feedback showed that I performed at an unsatisfactory level in anatomy
So what?
How did you feel at the time? What was important about it? How do this relate to your overall development or learning? I was not surprised by my performance in this part of the exam, as I had found the anatomy questions hard. I don't think my revision notes were concise enough. I also have realised that I work better with diagrams and drawings to help me visualise the anatomy, so I need to use these more.
Now what?
List your goals, keeping them as specific as possible. • Condense my revision notes and use illustrated flash cards • Give myself plenty of time to cover each topic twice before the exam • Test my understanding when I am revising
How will you determine when this goal has been met?
Think about if the goal is achievable. How can you measure this goal? I will reassess my progress in the run up to the exam, but ultimately, I will know if I have met my goal when the next exam results are released. My aim is to improve to "satisfactory" in anatomy
What hurdles or challenges exist to you achieving this goal and how would you manage them?
What strategies can you put in place to manage possible challenges? How realistic is your goal? To save time drawing flashcards I will research if good quality illustrated anatomy flashcards exist that I can purchase I will use a revision timetable to identify my aims for the week ahead. Daily timetables do not work well for me but I find I am able to set and meet weekly goals when I allow for some flexibility day to day.
When do you expect to have completed this goal? By the next exam
What have you learned from this process that will aid your future learning? That I need to use visual learning aids for more complex or three-dimensional concepts. Making sure that I have access to these learning resources will help me be better prepared for the exams and will mean that I have a greater understanding of the topic.

Fig. 5.4 An example of a goal-setting template (adapted from the authors institution) incorporating elements of the What? So What? Now What? And SMARTER goals approaches (Borton 1970, Doran 1984)

Table 5.6 The key benefits of coaching

Benefits of coaching
One-to one Equal partnership Short encounters Prospective focus Developing specific goals or skills Supportive Giving and receiving feedback

Table 5.7 The GROW coaching model [17]

Setting **G**oals	What does the student want to achieve? How will they know when they have achieved it?
Assessing the current **R**eality	What is the context around their goal? What is currently stopping them from meeting the goal? What have they achieved so far?
Develop **O**ptions	What different courses of action could they take? Are there potential benefits to each of these?
Establish a **W**ay forward	What particular strategy have they chosen?

Coaching can be utilised in a variety of settings. Using a coaching model can be helpful when giving students feedback after a patient encounter, as it can be a useful way for students to reflect on their performance. It is a strategy that can be utilised by academic advising, which is explored further in the following section.

5.4.2 Academic Advising

Academic advising is an evolving field, and there is some debate in the literature about its philosophy and theoretical underpinnings [18–20]. Academic advising is about supporting learning, and can enhance the student experience [21, 22]. This is via structured meetings that occur at intervals between a student (advisee) and an advisor who understands the student's programme of study. It can help improve the academic progress of students and help them to achieve their personal development goals. It also encourages students to develop their reflection and goal-setting skills. Academic advisors normally have a sustained relationship with their advisees during the programme of study. Regular meetings with advisees can help students to reflect on their studies and enhance their learning and self-critical awareness skills. They also can nurture student engagement and provide a personal connection to the programme and enhance student belonging [21]. Where possible it is sensible to embed academic advising into the curriculum and timetable meetings to encourage student engagement. The academic advisor may act as a coach who may supports students during their personal development and guide them in developing insight that they may need to become reflective professionals [23, 24, 25]. Academic advisors should receive training on how to guide the students through their academic and personal development goals [26, 27].

Academic advising should:
- Be embedded in the curriculum.
- Be compulsory to students.
- Address non-participation.
- Be relevant to students.
- Be collaborative.
- Consider utilising a coaching philosophy.

The academic advisor–advisee relationship is reciprocal. It will be most successful if students engage with the process and if their advisors provide appropriate support and guidance. The academic advising process is ongoing throughout the period of study. Meetings can be used to discuss potential goals and agree priorities, and to review the outcomes of earlier goals. In between meetings, students are expected to reflect on their goals and work towards achieving them by implementing the appropriate learning strategies [28].

5.5 Conclusion

In healthcare, change is a certainty. Some elements of current dental curricula will be out of date in 15 years. As dental teachers, we can prepare our students for the changing landscape of dentistry that they will spend their working lives in, by supporting them to develop their reflection and goal-setting skills as they become self-directed in their learning. Dental teachers can help students acquire the skills they need to be self-directed learners throughout their careers, using the tools discussed in this chapter.

Competing Interests The authors have no conflicts of interest to declare that are relevant to the context of this chapter.

References

1. GDC. Enhanced CPD guidance. London: General Dental Council: 20; 2019. Available via GDC. https://www.gdc-uk.org/education-cpd/cpd/enhanced-cpd-scheme-2018 Enhanced CPD guidance for dental professionals. Accessed 27 Nov 2024
2. ADA (2023) Principles of ethics & code of professional conduct, American Dental Association, Council on Ethics, Bylaws and Judicial Affairs: 26. Available via ADA https://www.ada.org/about/principles/code-of-ethics ADA code of ethics. Accessed 27 Nov 2024.
3. Houle CO. The inquiring mind. Madison: University of Wisconsin Press; 1961.
4. Tough AM. Learning without a teacher. A study of tasks and assistance during adult self-teaching projects. Toronto: Ontario Institute for Studies in Education; 1967.
5. Knowles MS. Self-directed learning: a guide for learners and teachers. New York: Association Press; 1975.
6. Hammond M, Collins R. Self-directed learning: critical practice. London: Routledge; 1991.
7. Gavriel J. Self-directed learner—the three pillar model of self-directedness. Boca Raton: CRC Press; 2015.
8. Garrison DR. Self-directed learning: toward a comprehensive model. Adult Educ Q. 1997;48(1):18–33.

9. O'Neill PA. Problem-based learning alongside clinical experience: reform of the Manchester Curriculum. Educ Health (Abingdon). 1998;11(1):37–48.
10. Poikela E, Nummenmaa A. Understanding problem-based learning. Tampere: University Press; 2006.
11. Rothman AI. Problem-based learning—time to move forward? Med Educ. 2000;34(7):509–10.
12. Loyens SMM, Magda J, Rikers RMJP. Self-directed learning in problem-based learning and its relationships with self-regulated learning. Educ Psychol Rev. 2008;20(4):411–27.
13. Grow GO. Teaching learners to be self-directed. Adult Educ Q. 1991;41(3):125–49.
14. Borton T. Reach, touch and teach: student concerns and process education. New York: McGraw-Hill Paperbacks; 1970.
15. Locke EA, Latham GP. Building a practically useful theory of goal setting and task motivation: a 35-year Odyssey. Am Psychol. 2002;57(9):705–17.
16. Doran GT. There's a SMART way to write management's goals and objectives. J Manag Rev. 1984;70:35–6.
17. Alexander G, Renshaw B. Supercoaching: the missing ingredient for high performance. London: Random House Business; 2005.
18. Wilson EA, Perman JA, Clawson D. Pearls for leaders in academic medicine. New York: Springer; 2008.
19. Drake JK, Jordan P, Miller MA. Academic advising approaches strategies that teach students to make the most of college. San Francisco: Jossey-Bass; 2013.
20. Burton SL. The debate begins: the rise of alternate perspectives in academic advising theory. NACADA J. 2016;36(1):3.
21. Thomas L, Hockings C, Ottaway J, Jones R. Independent learning: student perspectives and experiences. York: Higher Education Academy; 2015. p. 1–56. Available via Advance HE. https://www.advance-he.ac.uk/knowledge-hub/independent-learning-student-perspectives-and-experiences independent_learning_final. Accessed 24 Nov 2024
22. Thomas L, Hill M, O'Mahony J, Yorke M. Supporting student success: strategies for institutional change. What works? Student retention and success programme. London: Paul Hamlyn Foundation, Higher Education Academy, Action on Access; 2017. p. 1–32. Available via Advance HE. https://www.advance-he.ac.uk/knowledge-hub/supporting-student-success-strategies-institutional-change what_works_2_-_full_report. Accessed 24 Nov 2024
23. Tekian A, Jalovecky M, Hruska L (2000) A quantitative assessment of "At Risk" students and medical school performance: the importance of adequate advising and mentorship. Annual meeting of the American Educational Research Association. New Orleans: 1–10. 24–28 April 2000.
24. Schrubbe K. Mentorship: a critical component for professional growth and academic success. J Dent Educ. 2004;68:324–8.
25. Koole, S., V. Christiaens, J. Cosyn and H. De Bruyn (2016). Facilitating Dental Student Reflections: Using Mentor Groups to Discuss Clinical Experiences and Personal Development. Journal of dental education 80: 1212-1218.
26. Hendricson W, Kleffner J. Assessing and helping challenging students: why do some students have difficulty learning? J Dent Educ. 2002;66:43–61.
27. Al-Ansari A, El Tantawi M, Abdelsalam M, Al-Harbi F. Academic advising and student support: help-seeking behaviors among Saudi dental undergraduate students. Saudi Dent J. 2015;27:57–62.
28. Crookston BB. A developmental view of academic advising as teaching. J Coll Stud Pers. 1972;13:12–7.

Modelling and Simulation in Dental Education

6

Sabu Thomas, K. P. Jayachandran, Saju Joseph, and Taniya Rose Abraham

6.1 Introduction

The field of education is constantly evolving in response to rapid technological advancements. With the increasing globalisation of higher education and transnational collaborations, there is a growing expectation for institutions to maintain

S. Thomas (✉)
International and Interuniversity Centre for Nanosciences, Mahatma Gandhi University, Kottayam, Kerala, India
e-mail: sabuthomas@mgu.ac.in

K. P. Jayachandran
School of Nanoscience and Nanotechnology, Mahatma Gandhi University, Kottayam, Kerala, India

School of Pure and Applied Physics, Mahatma Gandhi University, Kottayam, Kerala, India

S. Joseph
School of Nanoscience and Nanotechnology, Mahatma Gandhi University, Kottayam, Kerala, India

T. R. Abraham
School of Energy Materials, Mahatma Gandhi University, Kottayam, Kerala, India

R. M. Baiju, S. Thomas (eds.), *The Dental Teacher*,
https://doi.org/10.1007/978-3-032-07551-2_6

high educational standards. In this regard, dental education requires the acquisition of fine motor skills, which must be systematically developed during preclinical training. However, research indicates that students often experience significant stress when transitioning from preclinical instruction to real clinical procedures [1]. To bridge this gap and better prepare students, educators have long relied on simulation-based learning as an effective instructional strategy [2]. The application of simulation in dental training has a long history, dating back to the eighteenth century when restorative procedures were practised on extracted teeth. Over time, advancements led to the introduction of phantom head simulators in the early twentieth century, providing students with more realistic training models [3]. Modern dental education institutions continue to integrate mannequins and simulation labs, where students refine their skills using artificial teeth under guided supervision [4].

Recent breakthroughs in virtual reality, robotics, and haptic technologies have further revolutionised dental simulations, offering immersive and interactive training experiences [5]. These innovations not only enhance skill development but also create a smoother transition from simulated environments to real clinical settings. Today, simulation-based training encompasses a range of dental procedures, including restorative dentistry, endodontics, periodontal assessments and implant placements [6].

Despite these advancements, traditional preclinical training often lacks exposure to common clinical variations such as drifting, supra-eruption and tilting due to arch integrity loss. Simulation-based approaches can address these gaps by incorporating problem-based learning techniques, allowing students to practise the clinical procedures in a controlled environment [7]. Additionally, the latest haptic virtual reality simulators provide sensory feedback, replicating realistic patient conditions, including mandibular movements and soft tissue interactions [8].

By integrating advanced simulation models into dental education, institutions can enhance students' practical skills, critical thinking and confidence, ensuring they are well-equipped for clinical practice. As technology evolves, refining simulation techniques will be essential in shaping the future of dental education and training. Dentistry has undergone significant advancements with the continuous integration of cutting-edge technologies, enhancing both education and clinical practice. The incorporation of computer-assisted tools, such as artificial intelligence (AI), virtual reality (VR) techniques and 3D printing, has advanced dental education by providing immersive and hands-on learning experiences. These technological innovations not only improve students' practical skills but also contribute to more precise diagnosis and treatment planning. As the demand for technologically skilled dental professionals grows, educational institutions are increasingly adopting simulation-based training methods to bridge the gap between theoretical knowledge and clinical practice [9] (Fig. 6.1).

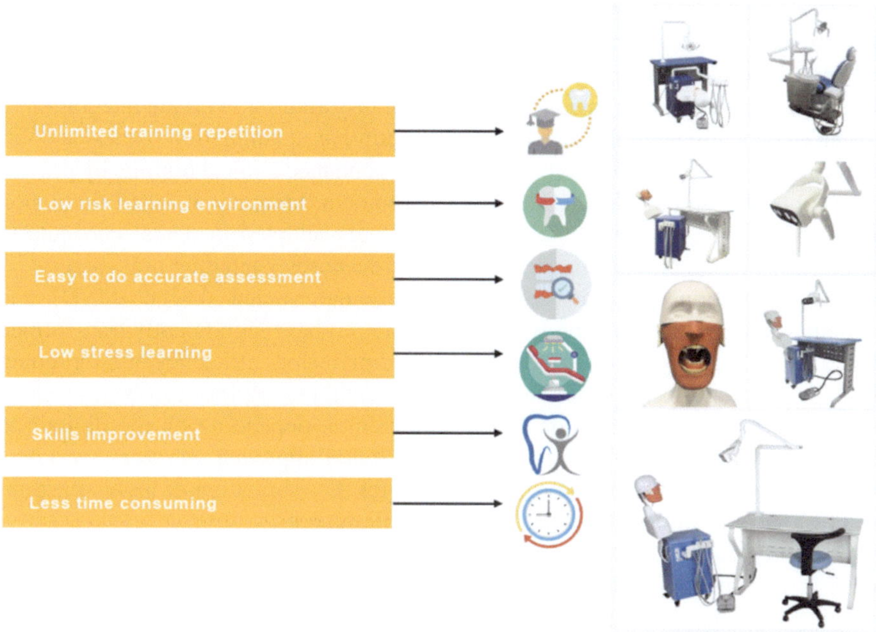

Fig. 6.1 Advantages of modelling and simulations in clinical practices of dental education

6.2 Technological Evolutions in Dental Practices

The integration of simulations in dental education dates back to 1894 when Oswald Fergus introduced the first phantom head simulator using a metal rod and two brass jaws. His assertion that students should not be allowed to practise on real patients without first achieving a certain level of competency underscored the necessity of simulation-based training [10]. Over a century later, simulation has become an essential component of dental curricula. However, traditional teaching methods continue to dominate, and the full potential of simulation remains underutilised [11].

Whilst advancements in simulation have transitioned from mechanical models to digital technologies, numerous questions persist regarding their effectiveness and implementation. The major concerns include the evidence supporting digital simulation, the optimal timing and integration within curricula, the level of exposure required for clinical competency, and its impact on patient safety [12]. Additionally, defining benchmarks for simulation effectiveness remains a critical challenge.

As the COVID-19 pandemic significantly disrupted healthcare education, it further emphasised the necessity of digital simulation as a resilient training tool [13]. The pandemic has accelerated the shift towards virtual and remote learning, underscoring the need for innovative and effective simulation technologies in dental education. This report aims to serve as a valuable resource for educators seeking to enhance dental training in a post-pandemic world. Traditional teaching methods in dental education are undergoing a significant transformation with the integration of advanced educational tools, including mannequin-based simulation models and virtual reality. These emerging technologies aim to enhance clinical training by providing a controlled and interactive learning environment. Mannequin-based simulation models [14] have, in particular, been increasingly adopted in dental curricula to facilitate hands-on practice in various dental procedures, including oral surgery.

The integration and advancements of computer-aided design (CAD) and computer-aided manufacturing (CAM) technologies have significantly transformed dental restoration processes, offering increased precision, efficiency and reproducibility. Laboratory-based CAM fabrication of dental restorations can be performed either in a dental laboratory or at a milling centre, depending on the digitalised design provided by the lab technician. This digital approach enhances workflow efficiency, minimises human error and allows for the fabrication of highly customised restorations tailored to patient-specific requirements.

Currently, CAD/CAM systems are widely utilised in dental practices and laboratories across the globe. These systems differ significantly in terms of their capabilities, accuracy, materials used and processing methods. Some systems are designed for chairside use, enabling same-day restorations, whilst others are laboratory-based, requiring additional processing steps before final delivery to the clinician. The advantages of CAD/CAM technology include improved fit and marginal adaptation of restorations, reduced fabrication time and the ability to use high-strength materials such as zirconia and lithium disilicate. However, challenges remain, including high initial investment costs, material limitations and the need for skilled operators to optimise design parameters and milling accuracy.

The CAD/CAM restorative digital workflow (Fig. 6.2) follows a structured sequence that includes digital impression acquisition, virtual design, milling or three-dimensional (3D) printing, and final adjustments before clinical placement. As advancements in digital dentistry continue to evolve, research is focused on

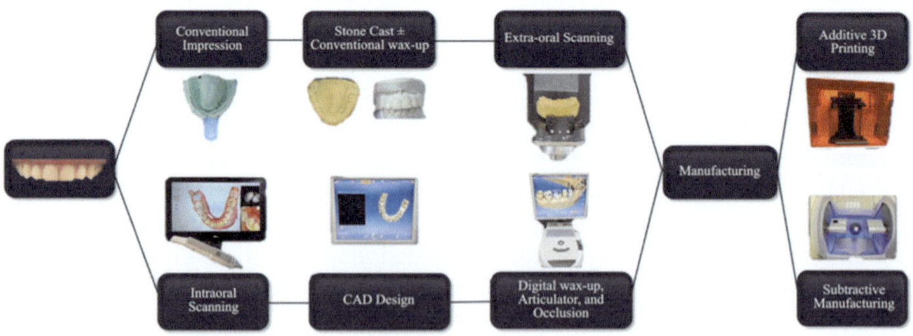

Fig. 6.2 The digital workflow of computer-aided design (CAD) and computer-aided manufacturing (CAM) (https://doi.org/10.7717/peerj.17793)

improving system efficiency, material properties and the integration of artificial intelligence to further enhance the automation and precision of dental restorations [15].

Simulation-based training has long been a part of dental education, providing the required skills students to develop clinical and practical skills before transitioning to patient care. However, recent advancements in virtual reality (VR) technology have introduced a new dimension to dental simulations, utilising computer-generated three-dimensional (3D) environments to enhance the learning experience. These VR-based medical simulations provide an interactive and immersive platform, bridging the gap between traditional mannequin-based simulation laboratories.

Several studies highlight the advantages of VR in dental education. Compared to conventional simulation techniques, VR-based training has been associated with greater learning efficiency, improved skill acquisition and objective, reproducible feedback mechanisms. Additionally, VR allows for unlimited practice opportunities, independent of faculty supervision, thereby extending training hours and enhancing cost-effectiveness for educational institutions. The ability to simulate complex procedures repeatedly in a risk-free setting further reinforces procedural confidence among students.

Despite its benefits, the adoption of VR in dental education is not without challenges. High initial setup costs, the need for specialised faculty training, and limited diversity in existing educational simulation programmes have been cited as barriers to widespread implementation. As the technology evolves, addressing these limitations will be necessary in optimising the role of VR in dental education. Ongoing research and technological advancements are expected to refine VR applications, making them more accessible and effective in preparing students for clinical practice [16].

6.3 Types of Simulations Used in Dentistry

All healthcare professions require a combination of theoretical knowledge from textbooks and lectures, as well as hands-on training to develop essential clinical skills. With an increasing focus on safety in medical and dental practices, the adoption of healthcare simulations has expanded significantly. In addition to conventional pre-clinical simulation labs, advanced technologies such as virtual reality with haptic feedback and life-like mannequins have been integrated into training programmes. These innovations aim to bridge the gap between theoretical learning and clinical application, ensuring that dental students acquire the necessary skills before performing real procedures. This chapter explores the latest advancements in simulation technologies, including those currently in use and those still in development, and examines their impact on dental education.

Various types of simulations are employed in dentistry, each designed to enhance different aspects of training. These include **mannequin-based simulations, virtual reality (VR) simulations, augmented reality (AR) simulations, haptic-based simulations, 3D-printed models for simulation, standardised patient simulations, and computer-assisted learning (CAL) simulations.**

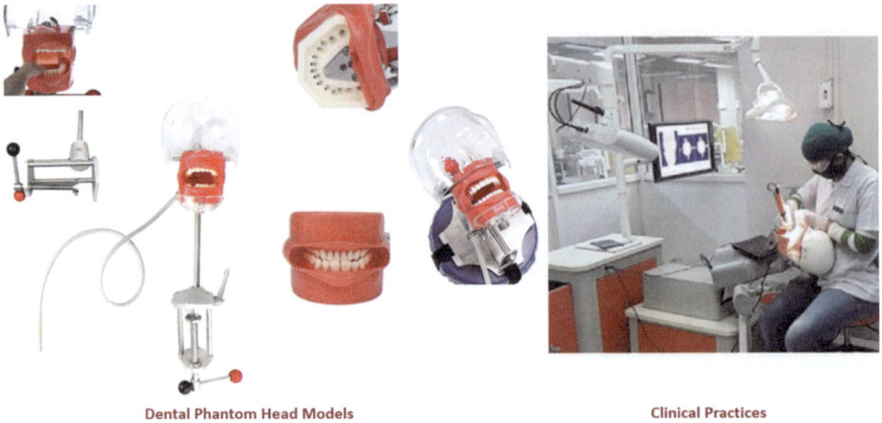

Fig. 6.3 Mannequin-based simulators and clinical practices

6.3.1 Mannequin-Based Simulations

Mannequin-based simulations play a crucial role in dental education by providing students with hands-on learning experiences in a controlled environment before transitioning to clinical practice. These simulations utilise life-like dental mannequins, also known as phantom heads, to replicate the human oral cavity, allowing students to practise various procedures with realistic anatomical features [17]. These simulators provide tactile feedback and are commonly used in pre-clinical training to familiarise students with basic hand skills. Mannequin-based simulators consist of a head model equipped with artificial teeth, soft tissue analogs, and an articulating jaw to mimic patient movements. Some advanced models include sensors to assess hand positioning, pressure application, and procedural accuracy. These simulators are widely used in pre-clinical training, helping students learn fundamental dental procedures such as cavity preparation, restorations, and prosthetic adjustments [18] (Fig. 6.3).

6.3.2 Virtual Reality (VR) Simulations

Recently, virtual reality (VR) simulations have been increasingly utilised in clinical dental practices as a supplementary tool to conventional skill training, providing students with hands-on experience before engaging with real patients. Unlike other medical disciplines, dental education requires a unique blend of theoretical knowledge, laboratory exercises and clinical practice. One of the primary challenges in this field is that acquiring theoretical knowledge demands strong spatial visualisation skills, whereas patient-centred training using conventional mannequin-based simulations often fails to replicate real clinical practices.

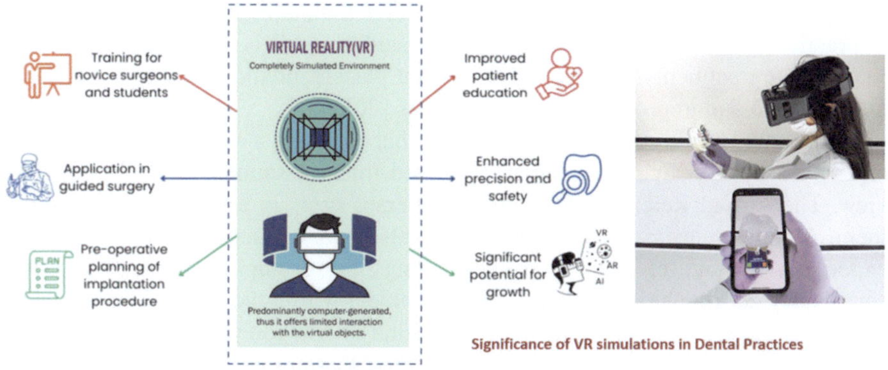

Fig. 6.4 Significance of virtual reality (VR) simulations in dental education

The clinical and preclinical training play a crucial role in refining fine motor skills, ensuring that dental students are well-prepared for professional practice. However, mastering the required competencies in dentistry is inherently difficult, necessitating repetitive training and extensive practise. The global outbreak of the novel coronavirus (SARS-CoV-2) in late 2019 significantly disrupted educational systems, imposing social distancing measures that affected traditional in-person teaching methods. As a result, the conventional one-on-one pedagogical model in dental education had to be replaced partially with digital and virtual alternatives to minimise student gatherings in enclosed environments. This shift has further accelerated the adoption of VR-based training tools in dental curricula.

Virtual reality (VR) is increasingly being recognised as an effective tool for training dental students, with its adoption steadily rising across dental institutions worldwide (Fig. 6.4).

VR technology creates a **computer-generated, immersive three-dimensional (3D) environment**, allowing users to interact with simulated clinical scenarios through specialised software [2]. By wearing a **head-mounted display (HMD)**, students can experience a **realistic and interactive setting**, engaging with virtual patients and environments in a way that closely resembles real-life experiences. This technology offers significant advantages in dental education by providing a **non-contact training platform**, enabling students to refine their clinical skills in a safe and controlled environment before transitioning to patient care. Also, VR platforms enable unlimited practice opportunities without the need for physical models [19].

6.3.3 Augmented Reality (AR) Simulations

In the field of dental technology, augmented reality (AR) simulations enable dentists to visualise and practice complex procedures using a virtual model of a patient's mouth. By overlaying digital information onto the real-world view through specialised AR glasses, practitioners can gain real-time insights into the treatment process.

This technology serves as a valuable preoperative tool, allowing dentists to perform a 'practice run' before conducting actual procedures. AR is particularly beneficial for intricate treatments such as dental implant placement and oral surgery, enhancing precision and improving patient outcomes [20].

Augmented Reality (AR) is a technology that enhances a user's perception of the real-world by overlaying computer-generated images, sounds, or data onto their view. The Virtual Reality (VR), which immerses users in a fully digital environment, AR integrates virtual elements into real-world settings, enriching the user's experience without replacing their surroundings. For example, AR-enabled glasses can display additional information about an object within the user's field of vision, offering a seamless blend of physical and digital interaction (Fig. 6.5).

In dental education, AR provides an interactive learning experience that enhances spatial awareness, depth perception and procedural precision. By offering layered visualisations of dental structures, AR enables students to examine internal anatomical details such as the placement of nerves and blood vessels without making an incision. This technology bridges the gap between theoretical knowledge and clinical application, allowing dental students to practise procedures such as root canals or implant placements in a risk-free, controlled environment. The ability to make mistakes, learn from them and refine techniques before working on actual patients makes AR an invaluable tool for modern dental training. It is also

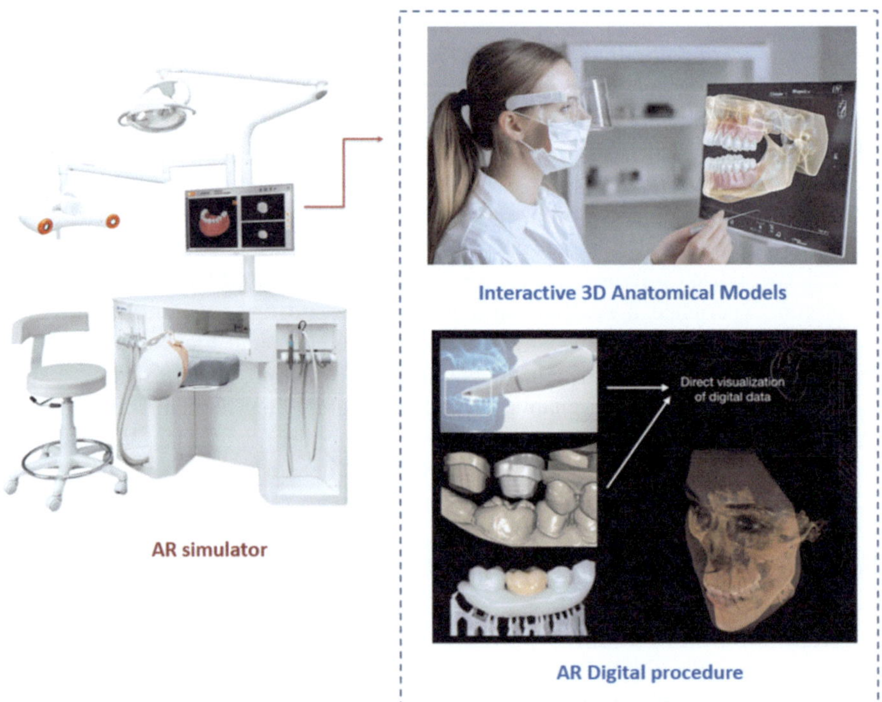

Fig. 6.5 Augmented reality (AR) simulation in dental education

applicable for procedural guidance, treatment planning and patient education, allowing students to visualise anatomical structures and simulate treatments in real time.

6.3.4 Haptic-Based Simulations

Haptic virtual reality simulation (HVRS) is a new technology in the field of teaching and learning operative dentistry [21]. Haptic-based simulations are an advanced technological innovation in dental education, providing students with a realistic sense of touch and resistance whilst performing virtual dental procedures. These simulations integrate force-feedback technology, allowing users to experience the texture, density, and pressure required for tasks such as tooth drilling, cavity preparation and root canal treatments. Unlike traditional simulation models, which rely on mannequins and physical dental models, haptic-based systems create interactive virtual environments where students can develop their manual dexterity and refine their clinical techniques.

The major significance of haptic simulations is their ability to offer repetitive, risk-free training, enabling students to hone their motor skills without the constraints of physical resources. These systems also provide real-time feedback, guiding learners through correct procedural steps and identifying errors instantly. As a result, students can practise various clinical techniques in a controlled setting, improving their precision and confidence before transitioning to real patient care.

Haptic technology is increasingly being incorporated into dental curricula worldwide, complementing virtual reality (VR) and augmented reality (AR) systems. By simulating lifelike clinical scenarios, haptic-based training tools bridge the gap between theoretical knowledge and hands-on practice, ultimately enhancing the overall learning experience in modern dental education. Compared to mannequin-based simulators, haptic-based dental simulators offer a more cost-effective alternative, as they do not require physical model replacements. Additionally, these simulators integrate haptic devices capable of measuring the forces exerted by trainees whilst interacting with a virtual patient's mouth. This feature enables real-time feedback, allowing for the detection of overly aggressive actions.

Several notable haptics based dental simulation techniques have been developed as follows:

- **Virtual reality dental training system (VRDTS):** This training system proposed by Novint Technologies in joint association with the Harvard School of Dental Medicine, this system focuses on cavity preparation. It simulates a variety of dental instruments—including a low-speed drill, explorer, carvers, carrier, and packer—along with amalgam material and a virtual molar containing enamel, dentin, caries, and pulp structures.
- **Iowa dental surgical simulator (IDSS):** A joint effort between the University of Iowa's College of Dentistry and the Graphical Representation of Knowledge

(GROK) Lab, this simulator allows users to experience different textures of enamel, healthy dentin and carious dentin whilst interacting with a virtual tooth.

- **3D dental:** Commercialised by SimuLife in 2002, this simulator provided tactile feedback to mimic real clinical sensations, such as caries probing, drilling, and cavity filling, using a virtual explorer or drill. However, this system is no longer available.
- **Haptically enabled dental simulator:** Designed by Montgomery et al. [22], this system combined high-resolution imaging techniques—including micro-CT scans, microgrindings and photographic images—to construct a detailed 3D virtual tooth. Users could simulate the tactile sensations associated with tooth preparation.
- **Volume-based dental simulator:** Developed by Kim and Park [23], this simulator was designed to train dental students in procedures such as dental probing, diagnosing carious lesions, performing drilling operations for cavity preparation, and filling cavities with amalgam. It utilised volume-based haptic rendering combined with polygonal mesh graphics for realistic visualisation (Fig. 6.6).

Whilst previous haptics-based dental simulators have effectively simulated restorative dentistry procedures such as cavity preparation and filling, they have not been designed to replicate periodontal treatments. In contrast, this haptics-based simulator is specifically developed for periodontics, a branch of dentistry where tactile perception plays a crucial role in both diagnosis and surgical procedures. Given the reliance on touch sensitivity in periodontal treatments, haptic technology is particularly well-suited for creating realistic training simulations in this field.

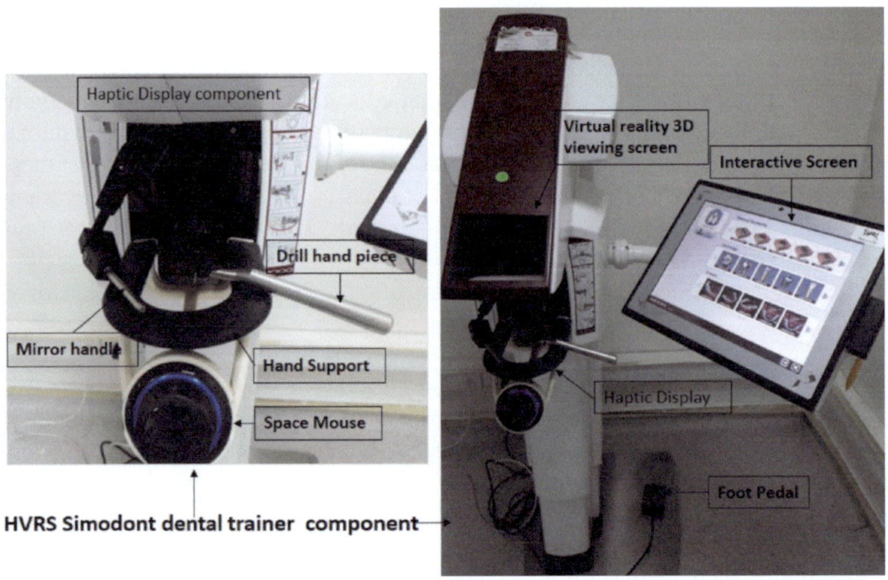

Fig. 6.6 Haptic virtual reality simulator (HVRS) simodont dental trainer [21]

6.3.5 3D-Printed Models for Simulation

Three-dimensional (3D) printing, known as additive manufacturing, offers a compelling alternative to extracted teeth and traditional dental models. 3D-printed teeth enhance educational accessibility whilst providing a highly realistic simulation of natural teeth, making them valuable for dental training and practice. The integration of 3D printing technology has significantly advanced various aspects of dentistry, including clinical, experimental and educational domains. Clinically, it has enabled the production of customised dentures, maxillofacial prostheses, crowns, bridges, orthodontic appliances, implants, and 3D-printed teeth. Beyond clinical applications, 3D-printed teeth are increasingly being used for educational purposes. Research indicates that incorporating these models enhances learner engagement and improves clinical skill development. These models allow students to practice complex procedures such as bone grafting, orthodontic treatments, and prosthetic fabrication in a realistic setting.

6.3.6 Computer-Assisted Learning (CAL) Simulations

Computer-Assisted Learning (CAL) has gained significant prominence over the past decade and is often referred to as Computer-Based Instruction (CBI), Computer-Aided Learning (CAL), or Computer-Aided Instruction (CAI). In this review, CAL is broadly defined as learning processes and environments that are supported by computers. A fundamental aspect of CAL is interaction, which occurs at multiple levels. At one level, students engage directly with digital content and learning materials, such as interactive simulations or virtual patients on a CD-ROM. Additionally, computers enable interactions between students and tutors, peer-to-peer communication, and collaboration within virtual learning communities. The following outlines how CAL works:

6.3.6.1 Role of CAL in Dental Education

Computer-Assisted Learning (CAL) has proven to be an effective educational tool in dentistry, offering an interactive learning experience that integrates text, two-dimensional (2D) and three-dimensional (3D) images, videos, animations, sound, and personalised interactions. These programmes guide students through structured learning paths or allow them to explore topics independently based on their learning objectives. Many CAL programmes simulate real-life diagnostic scenarios, placing students in an interactive role as a dentist [24]. Their diagnoses are evaluated based on the information accessed, and some of these programmes are designed using the Problem-Based Learning (PBL) approach.

6.3.6.2 Available CAL Programmes in Dentistry

A wide range of CAL programmes exists, varying in complexity from basic tutorials to advanced diagnostic simulations. These programmes have been assessed scientifically with varying degrees of success, primarily focusing on diagnosis and decision-making. Some evaluated CAL programmes are available in the following dental fields:

- **Anatomy**
- **Radiology**
- **Orthodontics**
- **Prosthodontics**
- **Periodontology**
- **Implantology**
- **Endodontics**
- **Trauma management**

6.3.6.3 Practical Applications of CAL

The practical applications of CAL are significant in learning how to chart the teeth. Many students struggle with differentiating both sides of the mouth when transferring information into charts. A specialised CAL programme was developed to display lesion images and allow students to practice entering data into an electronic record. Evaluations showed that students using this digital approach performed 80% better in pre- and post-tests, compared to only a 39% improvement in the control group.

CAL is also valuable in pre-clinical education, particularly in training students on tooth preparation for fillings and crowns. Existing software tracks and analyses students' preparations in real time, generating three-dimensional (3D) visualisations of their work. These models enable students to review and refine their techniques, enhancing their overall learning experience. These simulations use artificial intelligence (AI) and adaptive learning algorithms to provide personalised feedback and assessment.

6.4 Emerging Importance of Simulation in the Dental and Medical Healthcare

To put the different ways of teaching into context, there are a lot of different needs and problems that come up when trying to prepare dental and medical students for professional work. The different types of modern simulations used in healthcare education and how important they are becoming in getting dentists and medical students ready for professional practice will be discussed. When these new graduates first start working, their standards are different from those of clinicians in the service sector. The year before starting work is still a time of stress and getting used to things. In addition to having the right information and skills, practice is also needed to learn how to think and make decisions. Students in medicine and dentistry can learn a lot from practicing how to care for patients in real-life practice settings. These experiences are given through simulations in medical and dental schools to better connect theory with practice and make the change from being a dental or medical student to a practicing clinician easier. The main goal of this study is to find out how simulations can help dental and medical students improve their clinical judgment.

In order to better understand and implement the many tasks that fall under this category of learning strategy, it is important to examine the educational theories and frameworks that are pertinent to modern healthcare simulators. Whilst the social science literature will be cited, the primary emphasis will be on healthcare, dental, and medical education. An analysis will be conducted with a focus on the theories whose concepts offer the best frameworks for designing and carrying out simulations that help students develop the skills necessary to become registered dental, medical, or healthcare practitioners. Despite the emphasis on dentistry, medicine, and healthcare education, many students in these fields might benefit from the evaluated learning theories for simulation-based education. Additionally, simulations as a form of ongoing clinical education might be relevant.

6.5 Patient Safety and Simulation

The use of simulation as a teaching tool in dental and medical healthcare education has grown in recent years, either to support qualified clinicians in continuing their professional development or to prepare medical and dental professionals, as well as students, for practice. There is increased competition and challenges in obtaining student clinical placements, alongside the need to reduce medical errors and enhance patient safety and the quality of treatment. Simulations assist medical and dental professionals in preparing for their careers in various ways. Through these modern learning techniques, special focus is paid to the formation of clinical judgment.

A wide variety of patient care experiences cannot always be guaranteed through clinical practicum for medical and dental professionals. The time, location, and suitable opportunities for supervised practice all influence the kind of experience gained. Dental and medical professionals are more likely to have experienced desirable clinical events and to understand the care and patient management required of them by being exposed to fundamental patient care scenarios within simulation environments. Redesigning patient care procedures from a systems and personal perspective, especially through education and simulation techniques, has received a lot of attention. To improve the technical, behavioural, and collaborative abilities within the dental and medical fields, specific programmes and courses with integrated patient safety objectives were created and implemented [25, 26].

Globally, health-related simulation and clinical skills centres have appeared in hospital and educational settings, allowing human manikins to be used to model patient care scenarios in a real-world clinical setting. One of the main justifications for investing in such environments and resources is the way that simulations offer the chance to learn from mistakes without endangering patients. This is a conscious shift away from learning 'on the patient' and practicing tasks for the first time to the secure confines of a simulation lab, partly because of more realistic technology and a more aware public that is unwilling to be 'experimented on'.

Participants are given the chance to receive feedback from experienced dental and medical healthcare professionals after the simulation, which encourages them to reflect on their practice and find ways to improve it. The dental and medical communities must modify their culture from one that values secrecy and self-preservation to one that values transparency and openness to change in order to ensure the safety of their patients. Changing the culture of practice in the dentistry and medical disciplines involves ensuring confidentiality within simulated situations that mimic participants' practices [27–29].

6.6 Conclusion

The integration of simulation technologies in dental education has significantly improved the quality of training, allowing students to gain hands-on experience without the risks associated with live patient interactions. As technology advances, the continued development of these simulation methods will further enhance dental training, making it more efficient, immersive and widely accessible.

References

1. Divaris K, Barlow PJ, Chendea SA, Cheong WS, Dounis A, Dragan M, et al. The academic environment: the students' perspective. Eur J Dent Educ. 2008;12(1):120–30.
2. Perry S, Bridges SM, Burrow MF. A review of the use of simulation in dental education. Simul Healthc. 2015;10(1):31–7. https://doi.org/10.1097/SIH.0000000000000059.
3. Chowdhury CR, Khatri ML, Gopinath V, Rai R. Evolution of dental simulators in preclinical training: a historical perspective. J Dent Educ. 2021;85(9):1093–100.
4. Kneebone R. Simulation in surgical training: educational issues and practical implications. Med Educ. 2003;37(3):267–77.
5. Wierinck E, Puttemans V, Swinnen S, van Steenberghe D. Effect of augmented visual feedback from a virtual reality simulation system on manual dexterity training. Eur J Dent Educ. 2011;15(2):77–83.
6. Murbay S, Neelakantan P, Chang JWW, Yeung S, Bassir SH. Evaluating the effectiveness of haptic simulation in preclinical operative dentistry training: a meta-analysis. J Dent Educ. 2020;84(10):1056–66.
7. Ali K, Tredwin C, Kay EJ, Slade A. Problem-based learning in dental education: a review of the literature. Eur J Dent Educ. 2021;25(1):120–9.
8. Al-Saud LM, Mushtaq F, Allsop MJ, Culmer PR, Mirghani I, Yates E, Manogue M. Feedback and motor skill acquisition using a haptic dental simulator. Eur J Dent Educ. 2017;21(4):e101–6.
9. Economic Times (2023) The future of dental education in India: Incorporating new technologies. Retrieved from Economic Times.
10. Fergus O. Introduction of the phantom head simulator in dentistry. London: Dental Academy Press; 1894.
11. Smith J, Jones M. Advancements in dental education: simulation and traditional pedagogy. J Dent Res. 2019;45(2):89–102.
12. Brown R, et al. Digital simulation in clinical training: effectiveness and challenges. Int J Dent Educ. 2020;12(4):233–47.
13. Jones T, et al. Impact of COVID-19 on dental education and the role of digital simulation. Healthcare Educ J. 2021;15(3):178–95.

14. Taysi AE, et al. Evaluation of the efficacy of a simulation model used in oral and maxillofacial surgery education. BMC Med Educ. 2024;24:310. https://doi.org/10.1186/s12909-024-05307-3.
15. Zhang Y, Xu H, Lin C, Sun J, Li X. Artificial intelligence in digital dentistry: applications and future trends. Int J Oral Sci. 2021;13(1):26–39.
16. Lee T, Chen Y. Future prospects of virtual reality in oral surgery training. Clin Oral Investig. 2023;27(1):56–69.
17. Lavanya SH, Kalpana L. Mannequin-based simulation as an educational tool for learning injection techniques: medical students' view points. Int J Basic Clin Pharmacol. 2018;7(5):882–7. https://doi.org/10.18203/2319-2003.ijbcp20181629.
18. Singh V, Vidya B, Jameela RV, Bipinchandra LN, Bordoloi P, Srivastav M. The impact of virtual reality-based simulation training on dental students' clinical skills and confidence. J Pharm Bioallied Sci. 2024;16(Suppl 4):S3740–2. https://doi.org/10.4103/jpbs.jpbs_1218_24. Epub 2024 Nov 19. PMID: 39926724; PMCID: PMC11805292
19. Pottle J. Virtual reality and the transformation of medical education. Future Healthc J. 2019;6(03):181–5. https://doi.org/10.7861/fhj.2019-0036.
20. Lai P-L, Liu C-T, Po-Sung F, Chen J-H, Lan T-H, Wang J-C, Hung C-C. Achieving new excellence in an augmented reality dental education system. J Dent Sci. 2024;19(Suppl 2):S136–42., ISSN 1991-7902. https://doi.org/10.1016/j.jds.2024.07.023.
21. Farag A, Hashem D. Impact of the haptic virtual reality simulator on dental students' psychomotor skills in preclinical operative dentistry. Clin Pract. 2022;12:17–26. https://doi.org/10.3390/clinpract12010003.
22. Montgomery K, Herbranson E, Brown P. A haptically enabled dental simulator. In: MMVR 13, studies in health technology and informatics. Amsterdam: IOS Press; 2005.
23. Kim L, Park SH. Haptic interaction and volume modeling techniques for realistic dental simulation. Vis Comput. 2006;22:90–8.
24. Rendas AP, Rosado Pinto P, Gamboa T. A computer simulation designed for problem-based learning. Med Educ. 1999;33:45–54.
25. Higgins D, Hayes M, Taylor J, Wallace J. A scoping review of simulation-based dental education. MedEdPublish. 2016;27(9):36. https://doi.org/10.15694/mep.2020.000036.1. PMID: 38058871; PMCID: PMC10697570
26. Chowdhury H, Alam F, Mustary I. Development of an innovative technique for teaching and learning of laboratory experiments for engineering courses. Energy Procedia. 2019;160:806–11.
27. Elme L, Jørgensen ML, Dandanell G, Mottelson A, Makransky G. Immersive virtual reality in STEM: is IVR an effective learning medium and does adding self-explanation after a lesson improve learning outcomes? Educ Technol Res Dev. 2022;70(5):1601–26. https://doi.org/10.1007/s11423-022-10139-3.
28. Romancenco A, Saratila I, Ababii I, Rojnoveanu G, Dandara O, Spinei L. Bridging theory and practice: enhancing medical education through simulation-based training methods. Mold J Health Sci. 2024;2(11):68–73. https://doi.org/10.52645/MJHS.2024.2.09.
29. Elendu C, Amaechi DC, Okatta AU, Amaechi EC, Elendu TC, Ezeh CP, Elendu ID. The impact of simulation-based training in medical education: a review. Medicine (Baltimore). 2024;103(27):e38813. https://doi.org/10.1097/MD.0000000000038813.

Clinical Teaching

7

R. M. Baiju and K. Harikumar

7.1 Introduction

Clinical teaching begins at the bedside. The concept of medical teaching in the ward at the bedside started as early as 2000 years ago in Greece, where the father of clinical teaching Hippocrates, advocated the art [1]. Dentistry has traditionally looked up to Medicine for its existence and development in the initial formative years as a profession. Before the establishment of formal dental schools or structured training in universities, young aspiring dentists gained their knowledge and skills by observing and assisting their masters at the chairside. Sir William Osler, considered the father of modern medicine, has been the biggest proponent of bedside learning and he introduced the principle of learning by doing. According to Osler, medicine is learnt at the bedside more than in the classroom. In medical education, students visit patients, review their medical records and observe the teachers during their clinical interaction with patients until they formally qualify to literally practice the art. Whereas, dental students begin performing simple procedures during their studentship itself. Hence, dental students put on practice Osler's philosophy of learning by doing very early in their professional course curriculum compared to their medical counterparts.

Clinical teaching focuses on guided patient care, where every aspect of clinical care is guided and supervised by the clinical teacher. The close interaction of dental teachers and students in the clinical environment is paramount in developing clinical skills and professionalism among the students.

R. M. Baiju (✉)
Government Dental College, Kottayam, Kerala, India

Kerala University of Health Sciences, Thrissur, Kerala, India

K. Harikumar
Department of Periodontics, Government Dental College Kozhikode, Kozhikode, Kerala, India

R. M. Baiju, S. Thomas (eds.), *The Dental Teacher*,
https://doi.org/10.1007/978-3-032-07551-2_7

7.2 Learning by Observing Procedures

Clinical students generally observe a number of procedures several times before they can individually treat patients. Live clinical demonstration has its own limitations in a dental operatory setting due to multiple factors, including the number of students in the group, the detailed nature of the procedure and the inherent constraints of doing a procedure inside the oral cavity. Observing clinical procedures helps to refine necessary motor skills for a smooth delivery of clinical care. Observation of clinical procedures live reinforces standard desirable clinical protocols and promotes skill acquisition. Observation of a lengthy clinical procedure live, till end and in fine detail, is extremely labour intensive.

7.3 Role of the Clinical Teacher

Transformation from preclinical phase to clinical patient care is a landmark step in a professional dental student's journey. Dental students posted in various clinics observe, perform, refine and practice clinical skills and procedures under direct supervision. Clinical supervision and monitoring of dental students is not an easy job. Effective teacher is defined as 'someone who can impart his/her knowledge and skills successfully and able to bring about appropriate changes in knowledge, skills, attitudes and behaviours in his/her students' [2]. Effective clinical teaching requires direct supervision of the teacher, timely feedback and continuous communication with the student [3]. Good clinical teachers are skilful in guiding students' clinical work and bridging the gap between teaching and learning. Students acquire cognitive and meta-cognitive skills through six teaching methods namely modelling, coaching, scaffolding, articulation, reflection and exploration of the cognitive apprenticeship [4]. Of the 12 different roles that a teacher could play, the most important role in the context of clinical teaching is role modelling according to research reports [3]. The clinical teacher should strive to create clones capable of emulating his/her professional capabilities and, in due course, become better than him/her. Whilst the students perform clinical tasks independently, they should be allowed to do so and be provided with necessary *scaffolding* (support and guidance) when it is most needed. The teacher should encourage the student to *reflect* upon his/her clinical performance, including its strengths and weaknesses. The virtues of a clinical teacher that have received much recognition from students are punctuality, consistency, understanding and respect [5]. An enthusiastic, motivated and proactive teacher engages students through active participation and instils a desirable attitude and professional behaviour in them. Good teachers are not always born. Ordinary teachers can become exceptional teachers after continuous training. What is needed is a commitment and willingness to engage in lifelong learning.

7.4 Clinical Teacher Student Ratio

Clinical supervising staff/student ratio is an important factor that influences the effectiveness of clinical supervision. The reported ratios have been between 5:1 and 10:1; the generally accepted ratio is 8:1 [6]. In Cardiff University's community-based clinical teaching programmes, the ratio is 6:1, where dental students undertake total dental care within the premises of primary dental care [7]. When there are more students than this per clinical teacher, there will be a lack of availability of the teacher to supervise many students and provide timely feedback. This will result in poor learning outcomes and less-satisfied learners. Excessive workload will put a lot of stress on teachers as well [6]. Universities of international repute and academic centres of excellence recognise that clinical teaching is central to creating competent professionals and the quality of clinical teaching is highly dependent on staff strength and faculty training. A favourable teacher-student ratio and appropriate para-dental staff support are essential to imparting a quality learning experience to students [6]. According to a recent research report, students perceive that a lower teacher-student ratio would contribute to a better delivery of clinical instruction [3].

7.5 Teaching as a Unit

All clinical departments have multiple staff members at various career stages, depending upon their clinical experience, expertise and academic designations. They come from different cultural backgrounds and have different personal value systems, apart from varying teaching and clinical instructional abilities. It is highly important to teach the clinical subject as a team. Unless there is good, open communication among staff members and they work to achieve the departmental learning outcomes, the effectiveness of teaching will suffer. This is especially important in clinical sessions compared to lecture classes. Clinical teaching is a continuum and all teachers should be on the same page regarding the content planned and delivered. This is critical to ensure consistency in teaching. Clinical instruction should be based on mutually accepted, standard clinical protocols which are evidence-based and decided upon after adequate deliberations within the team. Department level staff meetings should be frequent and open discussions should happen regarding the progress of curriculum delivery and any changes to be made if needed. The senior members of the faculty should accept the role of mentors for newly joined staff and should provide all support and encouragement. Newly joined staff should be properly inducted to fit into the team and to make sure they deliver the right teaching content and in the right way.

7.6 Enabling Learning Environment

Making a professionally competent dentist out of a novice takes 3–4 years of continuous, rigorous training in a clinical environment. Students interact with many people during their clinical training, including their teachers, support staff, patients, bystanders and their peers. Good interpersonal skills and effective communication are essential for enjoying a memorable and effective learning experience. Learning happens better in a non-threatening environment. The role of the clinical teacher is paramount in ensuring an enabling learning environment, as students feel free to try new things in a safe, confident and supervised environment. Clinical instructors on duty have to be available, accessible, and approachable and willing to clarify doubts raised by students. The most important person in a student's clinic is the student and not the teacher or even the patient. Focus should be on providing a valuable learning experience to the students, utilising the care provided to the attending patient. Whilst focusing on teaching, enough treatment may not be completely provided in a single appointment, but this is not negative as the student's academic interests are taken care of with the consent of the patient [8].

7.7 Fundamental Steps in Clinical Skills Training

Achieving clinical skills through repeated practice in pre-clinical laboratory or simulation labs and then on patients is the present-day norm in clinical training. Numerous skills may be listed that are essential for a professionally competent dentist. *Diagnostic skills*, or the ability to work up a patient and arrive at a probable clinical diagnosis, are widely recognised ability. Some dentists may be good with *procedural skills*, that is, performing clinical procedures with good hand-eye coordination and exquisite psychomotor abilities. Some others may possess exceptional *communication skills* that stand out in comparison to their psychomotor or clinical decision-making abilities. Clinical teaching sessions ideally are designed to hone all the above-mentioned skills. The students should improve their diagnostic skills, procedural skills and communication skills. There has to be a didactic session to teach background knowledge prior to any skill training session. This may be provided through a lecture for a large group or through a small group discussion. The criticality/feasibility matrix determines whether a simulated skills lab session is needed prior to clinical performance. Those skills that are high in criticality have to be taught and practiced in the simulation lab multiple times through the DOAP (Direct Observation, Assist, Performance) method prior to doing it on a patient. Those procedures that are high on feasibility can be introduced to students safely on patients in the clinic. Once in the clinic, the first fundamental step is a demonstration of the skill on a patient. The clinical instructor performs the procedure on the patient, whilst the students (ideally four or five maximum) observe from close quarters (Fig. 7.2). The teacher explains and demonstrates slowly so that the students can follow and learn. Students may assist the teacher and the teacher handholds the student in performance as the next step. Then the student performs under direct observation and monitoring. Formative feedback by the clinical teacher is crucial for the student to achieve competency in the skill. After several sessions of hands-on practice, the student develops the ability to perform the task independently (*shows how*). The ability to demonstrate learning, or 'shows how', is tested during clinical examination (Fig. 7.1). 'Shows how' is the outcome of learning in a competence-based education scheme (Fig. 7.2).

Fig. 7.1 Miller's pyramid of clinical competence

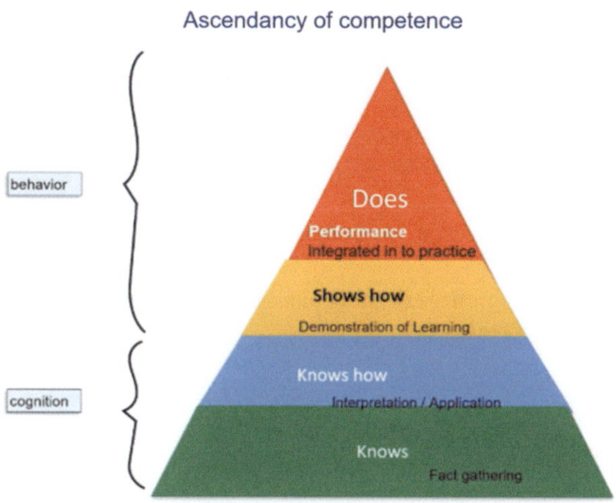

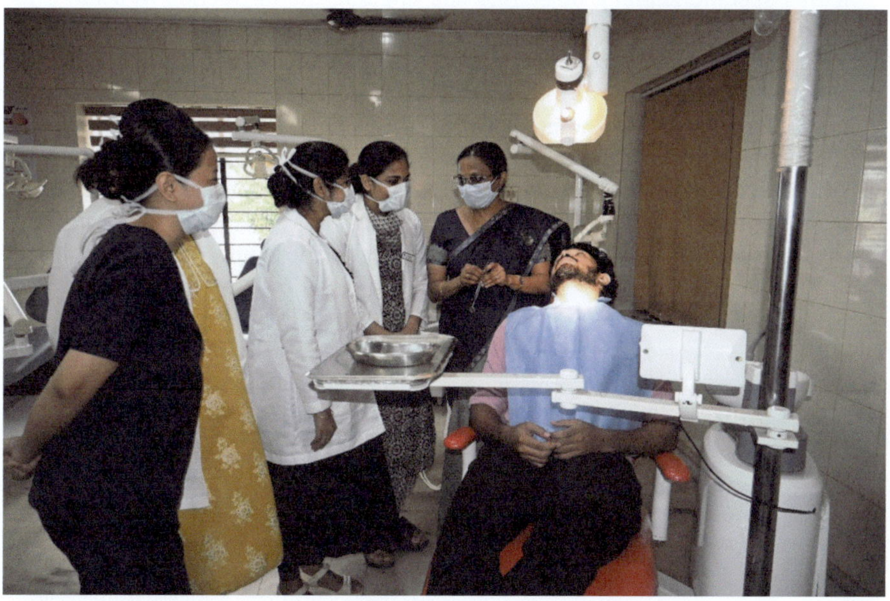

Fig. 7.2 Chairside clinical discussions for a small group with the patient in the chair

7.8 Knowing What to Teach in a Clinical Session

Both the clinical teacher and the students should be aware of what is taught in the upcoming clinical session. Each clinical session, irrespective of its duration or the seniority of the students, should ideally be based on specific learning objectives. As described in several other situations including research methodology, learning objectives should be SMART—*specific, measurable, achievable, relevant* and *time-bound.* Learning objectives can be better understood as having the following components:

A. Audience: target of the class.
B. Behaviour: demonstration by the learner about what has been learnt.
C. Condition: under what condition the learners are expected to perform what they have learnt.
D. Degree: extend of learning.

Learning clinical skills can be planned using on following objectives, similar to the ABCD criteria:

A. Audience: class of students.
B. Content: topic or skill.
C. Condition: given clinical situation.
D. Criteria: degree of learning as assessed on a scale.

Setting specific learning objectives and aligning the instruction to achieve the intended objectives is a highly effective and efficient approach to clinical teaching. The student should be informed about the learning objectives at the beginning of the session or well in advance of it. This will prepare them to receive the information with adequate preparation and homework.

Many effective teachers prepare a *teaching script*—an action plan of what, why, who, how and when of the session. Teachers early in their career can have a written script; accomplished teachers may have it in their mind.

The various factors that influence the chairside teaching are highlighted in Table 7.1.

Table 7.1 Factors influencing chairside teaching

1. One-to-one attention.
2. Non-threatening environment.
3. Facilitation to ask questions and clarify doubts.
4. Relevance of the session concerning the given patient.
5. Extend of student engagement in chairside sessions.
6. Teacher's experience and enthusiasm.
7. Informality of the learning environment.

7.9 The Importance of Feedback

Feedback by the clinical teacher is one important factor that drives learning. Providing timely feedback is a critical element in chairside teaching. Effective use of feedback is the backbone in the making of a competent dental professional, because feedback reinforces what needs to be done right and what should be corrected. There is a preferred manner for providing feedback effectively to students.

- *It has to be timely*: Do not delay it so that the incident is still fresh in memory.
- *It has to be specific*: Mention exactly what needs improvement or what exactly was done correctly.
- *It has to be descriptive*: Explain what was done right and what was not. Elaborate on what you intend to refine in the students' professional behaviour or clinical steps.
- *Feedback should be given with good intension*: to motivate and improve professional behaviour and not to criticise and demotivate.
- *Prioritise your comments*: Negative comments should come last. Always reinforce positive, desirable behaviour first.
- *Provide one-to-one feedback*: Avoid publicly delivering negative feedback.
- *Ask for the student's self-appraisal prior to giving your feedback*: Respond to it before offering feedback. Offer suggestions for improvement.
  In the competency based dynamic curriculum formative assessment is crucial and far important than summative assessment. As the attainment of competency is the outcome, effective feedback assumes great significance in the achievement of milestones and professional growth of the student in the dental school.

7.10 Clinical Teachers as Administrators

With increasing seniority, several administrative and other responsibilities may reduce the effective clinical teaching time. Senior staff may become integral members of the academic administration or the university, handling curriculum planning and development, or may handle academic staff training. Clinical teaching is a full-time job which requires continuous life-long learning and commitment. Additional job responsibilities that demand a lot of time and travel might negatively affect the clinical teacher's primary job due to the inability to allot sufficient time for teaching preparations and updating their knowledge base.

7.11 Patients as Teaching Resource

Patients are now better informed about their rights and privileges than ever before. It is going to be increasingly difficult to get patients as clinical material to teach students. New strategies are required to attract and retain patients in dental schools so that they can be utilised for clinical teaching. Appropriate liaison and specially designed care plan needs to be implemented to attract patients to ensure their availability in sufficient numbers at the right time in the clinical departments for the benefit of students posted there. Postgraduate programmes should not overshadow undergraduate teaching by utilising more patients and the bulk of staff time. An alternative learning opportunity is to set up advanced simulation laboratory. Although it is expensive, it is highly recommended to provide clinical simulation skill training to dental students. However, nothing can replace the real patient in a students clinic.

7.12 Changing Institutional Policies

Dental schools and universities now aim for rankings and accreditation to stay at the forefront and ensure adequate visibility in the educational arena. This is important in the new age for the existence and growth of the institution. Research, patents and publications are now highly valued as credentials of academic achievements. Dental teachers are required to take part in research and publishing as part of their career progress. Teaching should not become a low priority for schools or teachers at the expense of research. Institutional policies should recognise teaching as equivalent to research or other academic achievements like publishing.

7.13 Video as a Clinical Teaching Tool

Video has a wide range of applications as a teaching aid in clinical dental education. Video can be effectively utilised for simulation of clinical scenarios and for training of certain clinical or surgical skills [9, 10]. Video-Assisted Clinical Instruction in Dentistry (VACID) offers unobstructed magnified view of a clinical procedure being performed by the master clinician, either live or pre-recorded. VACID facilitates clinical instruction of concepts and skills [11]. Single or multiple ceiling-mounted cameras capture the images and display them a monitor, offering a clear magnified view of the procedure. Students can observe the procedures in the finest detail by pausing and playing the recorded video, keeping them engaged. Use of a head-mount camera has been suggested for clinical demonstration of dental procedures in an article by Chadwick et al. [12]. The head-mount camera sees what the demonstrator sees and in the way he or she sees it. The head-mount camera system was introduced by the Dundee dental school, where it was used for student demonstration as well as student assessment whilst he/she performs a procedure with the head-mount camera. It was concluded that this technique improved the level of detail observed by the students. It also improved the level of feedback.

Video demonstration is an invaluable toot in instruction of the affective domain, specifically for interpersonal training. Its unique characteristics make video a superior means for the development of communication and interpersonal skills training [13, 14]. Several studies by Kalwitzki et al. have reported the high student acceptance of video-based clinical teaching in undergraduate education [15, 16]. Watching videos created specifically for training dental students' could have a positive influence on their clinical behaviour in the future [16]. Other aspects of clinical behaviour that could be influenced by observance of clinical video-based instruction are non-verbal communication skills, infection control practices and ergonomics-complaint postures and positioning.

7.14 Learner-Centred Clinical Education

In an educational context, teaching has given way to learning. Students are now at the centre of the educational spiral. In the learner-centred clinical education, students, instead of being passive observers, take a proactive role in an educational encounter where patients are involved. When the learner takes the central role, teacher shifts to the role of facilitator, guiding the student through the learning process. The instructor guides instead of delivering. Actual experience and learning are integrated into experiential learning. A student dental clinic in a dental school is an outpatient education model. In the learner-driven educational encounter, the students and teacher engage in a collaborative intellectual exchange; the extent of it is determined by the involvement of the learner. The facilitator serves as a knowledge presenter rather than a knowledge source. The preceptor empowers the learner by promoting critical thinking and clinical reasoning.

7.15 SNAPPS

SNAPPS is a learner-driven-teacher-learner continuum. It is a six step structured learning encounter facilitated by the preceptor (teacher).

S—summarise briefly the history and clinical findings [17]

- The student obtains a history, conducts physical examination and presents a concise summary of findings.
- It should utilise about 50% of the time of the teaching.*
- Encounter, approximately 3 minutes.

N—narrow the differential to two to three relevant possibilities

- Student provides two to three possibilities of differential diagnosis. Students present their list.
- Teacher revise it if needed.

A—analyse the differential by comparing and contrasting the possibilities

- Student thinks loud in front of the preceptor. Explains his clinical reasoning and
- Suggest what is 'why' with respect to the patient's unique findings?

P—probe the preceptor/asks questions about difficulties or alternate approaches

- This helps the teacher to assess the student's knowledge base and prompts the preceptor for clinical pearls. The preceptor suggests things to be emphasised.

P—plan management of the patient's condition

- The student formulates and presents a treatment plan; teacher guides them with their knowledge and wisdom.

S—select a case-related issue for self-directed learning

- The student identifies a learning issue with the help of the preceptor and discusses the findings/observations from the learning issue with the teacher.

The SNAPPS model empowers the learner to give a case presentation based on their knowledge and understanding. The SNAPPS model is learner-driven and teacher-facilitated at the same time.

It is an adaptation of the traditional case history format. The unique features of SNAPPS are the active role of the learner, questioning the preceptor and the taking up of a relevant issue for self-directed learning. SNAPPS provides a brief but highly effective teaching and learning experience in the outpatient clinic. This model brings the learner and teacher together on the same platform as partners of this novel learning experience.

7.16 One Minute Preceptor

A lot of time is spent interviewing the patient and presenting the case in the dental clinic where students are posted to learn clinical cases. One Minute Preceptor (OMP) is a microteaching technique that tries to maximise the potential of the entire encounter between student and preceptor in a busy clinical schedule [18]. The teaching encounter lasts just over a minute, but the entire time is effectively used. OMP consists of five steps; each step is considered an individual teaching tool, which, when combined, forms an integrated approach to clinical teaching.

The five steps are as follows:

1. Get a commitment from the learner (*what do you think is the case?*)
2. Probe for the supporting evidence (*why do you think so?*)
3. Reinforce what was right.
4. Correct mistakes.
5. Teach the general rules (*teach clinical pearls*).

In the first step, the teacher tries to get a commitment from the learner regarding a case or a particular aspect of it. After the physical examination, when the preceptor asks the learner what he thinks about this case, it pushes him out of his comfort zone to make a commitment. This prompts the learner to process the gathered information to make a response. This is an adult learning experience. The right answer gets a positive reinforcement, and the wrong answer throws open an opportunity to teach. Suppose the learner is not in a position to give a commitment; the preceptor may ask further probing questions like ‘what other differential diagnosis would you consider?’ or ‘what do you think about his treatment?’

In the second step, it is important to explore the basis for the learner’s commitment. The preceptor here makes sure that it was not just a fancy guess but a logical response from processed information that the learner has gathered from the history and physical examination encounter. Here the clinical reasoning skill of the learner is tested.

In step three, what was done well will be reinforced. Words of appreciation and reassurance from the teacher will reinforce positive behaviour and skills in the learners.

It is equally important to tell them where they went wrong or what aspects need improvement. Hence, step four is vital. The preceptor has to be careful in avoiding extreme negative words like ‘bad’ or ‘poor’. Comments have to be precise and specific for effecting behaviour change. The criticism has to be a balance between constructive and positive. Also, shying away from providing corrective criticism is not a good habit from the preceptor as it impedes learning and progress of the student.

The last step is wisdom for future. The learner will take the information gained from the clinical experience to accurately generalise it to another similar situation in the future. The preceptor provides clinical pearls, so that when the learner encounters a similar situation later on, the principles learned from the clinical pearls can be effectively and rightly applied. It is important not to overgeneralise.

Managing time to teach is very critical in chairside teaching. An over-extended teaching session may delay patient care. Time management is entirely under the control of the teacher and OMP is a very effective strategy for clinical teaching in the busy environment of a dental clinic.

7.17 Challenges of Chairside Teaching/Common Problems

There are several challenges in providing chairside teaching sessions effectively in the student’s clinic on a routine basis. Time pressures deprive teachers of teachable moments. The clinical instructors work on a tight schedule with a predetermined work routine. If all of a sudden an interesting case is reported, the teacher may not be in a position to accommodate another session to show that case in between her already packed schedule. In certain centres where the student-teacher ratio is excessive, clinical teaching suffers. Many dental schools still follow the quota-based system of mandatory procedures to be performed in a prescribed quantity by the student. A lot of clinical time is lost in the attempt to finish the quota, depriving the intended chairside learning. If the teaching team does not follow a standardised, consensus-based procedure, clinical opinions may diverge, leading to chaos and confusion among students. Creative planning, anticipating the potential challenges, is essential to circumvent the deterrents and to fulfil what is to be achieved by the students at the end of the clinical posting.

7.18 Patient-Centred Approach in Chairside Learning

The most important person among the student-patient-teacher trio is the patient. The patient's expectations, values and needs are central to the clinical teaching environment. Adequate time should be spent for interviewing the patient to obtain relevant information regarding signs and symptoms. This is also the occasion to get data regarding his/her sociodemographic details, attitudes, demands and expectations. This information is critical in the treatment planning and prioritisation process. The ideal rules for a chair side instruction session are given in Table 7.2.

The traditional clinical learning model is specialist-directed, student-centred, and segmented. Each specialty clinical department acts as a stand-alone teaching station where specialty-centred treatment planning and care delivery are provided. Here the focus is on curriculum-centred procedures and numerical requirements. On the contrary, the comprehensive care model is considered more ideal and has a generalist role model. It is patient-centred education rather than student-centred. The patient management and evaluation are based on achievement of competence. The patient-centred model is fundamental in imparting training on cultural competence and social responsibility.

Emmanual and Emmanual have suggested four different physician-patient relationship models, namely paternalistic, informative, interpretive and deliberative models. Each model has its value according to individual clinical scenarios [19]. For example, in an emergency, a paternalistic model would be more suited as an incapacitated patient is saved by the treatment decisions of the treating physician who has considered the patients best interests. Out of the four models, the deliberative model has been considered the most suited on most occasions, as it augments patient autonomy, and adds care compassion and enables a patient-centred decision-making by a well informed and professionally supported patient. The traditional clinical dental training still has a bias towards a specialist doctored-led authoritarian approach of patient care [20]. On the other hand, a patient-centred clinical dental training environment strengthens the concept of informed consent, imparting a more mature educational experience to the clinical students. In a guided patient-centred approach, the student develops from novice through clinical competence to expertise [21]. Thus, all clinical teachers should be trained in the patient-centred

Table 7.2 Ideal rules for a chairside learning session

Brief the patient before the session about its purpose and their role.
Appropriately involve the patient to the extent possible.
Ensure equitable engagement of students.
Teach respect for patients' privacy and confidentiality.
At the end, learners summarise and the teacher concludes.
After the session, appreciate and thank the patient.

learning model. A good clinical teacher should always think in terms of the biopsychosocial model of patient care and act appropriately rather than adopting the medical model. This requires a thorough systems approach in designing the dental curriculum based on the patient-centred learning approach.

7.19 Conclusion

The profession of dentistry relies on various clinical skills. Chairside teaching is an integral instructional strategy in the competency-based dental education imparting the requisite skillsets to become a fully developed general dental practitioner. The clinical teacher should always consider to linking theory with practice. The adequate teacher-student ratio should be respected. Patients are important in a student clinic, but more important are the learning objectives of the students. Leaners should be taught to respect the privacy and confidentiality of the patients. The experienced clinical teacher serves as a role model and effectively manages time and resources to teach in their busy clinical time. Students learn best from a patient-centred approach and a generalist role model rather than a compartmentalised specialist role model of care. Above all, mentoring and role modelling are the finest virtues of clinical teaching that mould future dental professionals.

References

1. Aldeen AZ, Gisondi MA. Bedside teaching in the emergency department. Acad Emerg Med. 2006;13:860–6.
2. Khoo EM, Teoh KS. The effective teacher. Malays Fam Phys. 2007;2:123–4.
3. Shoaib LA, Safii SH, Naimie Z, Ahmad NA, Sukumaran P, Yunus RM. Dental students' perceptions on the contribution and impact role of a clinical teacher. Eur J Dent Educ. 2018;22(1):e26–34. https://doi.org/10.1111/eje.12252. Epub 2016 Dec 20. PMID: 27995730
4. Collins A, Brown JS, Newman SE. Cognitive apprenticeship: teaching the crafts of reading, writing, and mathematics. In: Resnick LB, editor. Knowing, learning, and instruction: essays in honor of Robert Glaser. Hillsdale: Lawrence Erlbaum Associates, Inc; 1989. p. 453–94.
5. Fugill M. Teaching and learning in dental student clinical practice. Eur J Dent Educ. 2005;9:131–6.
6. Martin N, Fairclough A, Smith M, Ellis L. Clinical educators' views on the quality of undergraduate clinical restorative dentistry in the UK and ROI. Eur J Dent Educ. 2011;15(4):216–22. https://doi.org/10.1111/j.1600-0579.2010.00659.x. Epub 2011 Jan 31. PMID: 21985205
7. Lynch CD, Llewelyn J, Ash PJ, Chadwick BL. Preparing dental students for careers as independent dental professionals: clinical audit and community-based clinical teaching. Br Dent J. 2011;210(10):475–8. https://doi.org/10.1038/sj.bdj.2011.383. PMID: 21617672
8. Harrington C, Robinson F, Mallery SR. Clinical teaching in dentistry: evaluating a clinical oral pathology rotation while looking to the future of dental education. J Dent Educ. 2023;87:1016–21. https://doi.org/10.1002/jdd.13206.
9. Chen MS, Horrocks EN, Evans RD. Video versus lecture: effective alternatives for orthodontic auxiliary training. Br J Orthod. 1998;25:191–5.
10. Robinson PB, Lee JW. The use of real time video magnification for the pre-clinical teaching of crown preparations. Br Dent J. 2001;190:506–10.

11. Fakhry A, Cooper SH, Slach N, Krenz TS. Video-assisted clinical instruction in dentistry. Overview and applications. Eur J Dent Educ. 2007;11:1–8.
12. Chadwick RG, Carena AP, Hunter B, Campbell K. Evaluation of a head mounted camera for clinical dental teaching. Br Dent J. 2008;204:93–6.
13. Gleber JM. Interpersonal communications skills for dental hygiene students: a pilot training program. J Dent Hyg. 1995;69:19–30.
14. Wepman BJ. Communication skills training for dental students. J Dent Educ. 1977;41:633–4.
15. Kalwitzki M. Acceptance of psychological teaching in paediatric dentistry by undergraduate dental students. Eur J Dent Educ. 1997;1:13–7.
16. Kalwitzki M, Rosendahl R, Go¨ ttle R, Weiger R. Acceptance of video-based teaching in paediatric dentistry by undergraduate dental students. Eur J Dent Educ. 2003;7:66–71.
17. Wolpaw TM, Wolpaw DR, Papp KK. SNAPPS: a learner-centered model for outpatient education. Acad Med. 2003 Sep;78(9):893–8. https://doi.org/10.1097/00001888-200309000-00010. PMID: 14507619
18. Irby D. The one-minute preceptor. Presented at the annual Society of Teachers of Family Medicine Predoctoral meeting, Orlando, FL; 1997.
19. Emanual EJ, Emanual LL. Four models of the physician patient relationship. JAMA. 1992;267(16):2221–16.
20. Eriksen HM, Bergdahl J, Bergdahl M. A patient-centred approach to teaching and learning in dental student clinical practice. Eur J Dent Educ. 2008 Aug;12(3):170–5. https://doi.org/10.1111/j.1600-0579.2008.00518.x. PMID: 18666899
21. Dreyfus SE. The five-stage model of adult skill aquisition. Bull Sci Tech Soc. 2004;24:177–81.

Principles of Assessment

8

K. Chandrasekharan Nair

8.1 Introduction

A good synonym of the term 'assessment' is 'evaluation' which was popularly used in educational circles, until recently. Other related terms are 'examination', 'test' and 'grading'. Assessment has a Latin root—'Assidere', which means to sit beside. In the Indian context, the ancient texts by the name 'Upanishad' has a meaning of 'sitting near the teacher'. Who are all those sitting beside in the process of education? It must be the teacher and the students. The teacher gets information from the student in smaller increments about what he knows and what he can do. The teacher can guide the student on the future course based on the information collected or deduced from the assessment process. In assessment, the student gets an opportunity to reflect or think aloud about what he knows and what he can do, which may help the student in his/her future course.

In the prevailing examination system, students are encouraged to showcase what they know and what they can do and the examiners do not intensively explore the areas in which the candidate is not proficient. The net effect is that the students go out with a notion that they know everything, which can stop their learning process and the principle of 'lifelong learning' is almost stalled.

8.2 The Purpose of Assessment

In the conventional context, assessment is used for the purpose of promotion from one class to the next. It is also used to screen students who seek admission for higher studies and to award degrees. At a higher level, assessment gives feedback to the

K. Chandrasekharan Nair (✉)
AECS Maaruthi College of Dental Sciences, Bangalore, India

Sree Sankara Dental College, Thiruvavanthapuram, India

R. M. Baiju, S. Thomas (eds.), *The Dental Teacher*,
https://doi.org/10.1007/978-3-032-07551-2_8

student on his achievement and the teacher also gets feedback whether the teaching methodology really worked or not. In the recent past, a huge quantity of research has been undertaken, and the understanding of assessment has changed perceptibly. The three dimensions of assessment are (1) assessment of learning, (2) assessment for learning, and (3) assessment as learning.

8.2.1 Assessment of Learning

In a classroom situation, assessment is usually done at the end of the term in the form of a test or examination where questions will be asked from the portions covered or studied. Here, the emphasis is given to summative assessment and the students are compared on the basis of the marks scored. Students are assigned a position in the class and the teacher's purpose is satisfied to that extent. However, there is no element of feedback or improvement included. There is widespread public support for this method of assessment and simultaneously the scepticism about increases on the fairness of the conduct of the assessment. Both formative and summative assessments have their own roles. A Facebook quote seems to clarify both forms of assessments: 'when the cook tastes the soup that is formative, when the guests taste the soup, that is the summative' (Bob Stake) [1, 2].

8.2.2 Assessment for Learning

Conventionally, assessment is considered an end process that decides the result (summative assessment). But it is not the real assessment because learning is a lifelong process which needs formative assessment characterised by providing feedback that encourages the learner to realistically appreciate not only the strengths but also the weaknesses. The feedback given at timely intervals improves learner outcomes, confidence and independence. Our aim is to create professionals who can look beyond the simplistic aim of 'only to get a degree' but to develop a professional who can understand the problems of the patient and who will readily provide appropriate treatment. Assessment for learning, stimulates the learner and simultaneously provides a feedback to the teacher on the effectiveness of the teaching also.

8.2.3 Assessment as Learning

Here, the student is encouraged to do a self-assessment on his learning and it is in the form of formative assessment. The student can seek help from his peers and the teacher only listens. Students can reflect, think and decide what to think about to find out solutions if they need any. In fact, this is the best time to sit beside the learner to understand the learner's thinking process. There is no threat of grades or comparison and hence the learner can self-evaluate freely and suggest their own corrections and adjustments. In other two forms of, the teacher has the role of key assessor, but in this form of assessment, the student assumes the role of key assessor [3, 4].

8.3 Short History of Assessment

Serious thinking on assessment in medical and dental education occurred towards the latter half of the twentieth century. Assessment was popularly known as an examination, which had the format of a written and clinical component aimed at determining the knowledge of the student. In dentistry, students were expected to perform select skills related to different specialities along with case presentation. The examination compulsorily included a 'viva' where the student had to exhibit analytical skills in a defensive mode. The examination or assessment could not claim a full representation of the curriculum, which is logically not possible.

Miller's pyramid should be mentioned in this context. Miller proposed the framework for clinical assessment. This consists of a pyramid with four levels. At the lowest level is knowledge (knows), above that are competence (knows how), performance (shows how) and action (does). Knowledge is no doubt important, but merely becoming knowledgeable will not make a learner proficient in the practice of dentistry. A professional should know how to use the knowledge acquired during the training period; then he or she will be considered as competent. The student should be able to show how to do what they have learned or perform. Clinical assessment in dentistry has included this for many years in the assessment system. The next is the crucial one where the graduate can successfully function in independent practice. This is the most difficult part of assessment (action) to be performed accurately and reliably.

The era of MCQs was ushered in by Kelly F. J. through his dissertation submitted to the Columbia University, New York, as early as 1915. He suggested this as a solution to avoid errors committed by many evaluators. The United States used this later in categorising army recruits during the World war I. Towards the end of twentieth century; MCQs were introduced to dental and medical education. Presently, the single best response type of MCQ is the most popularly used objective type test in screening dental and medical aspirants. There is only one correct answer and hence the objectivity remains unquestioned. In the evolution of assessment, Modified essay questions (MEQs) and Patient management problems (PMPs) are also popularly used for their high level of reliability [5].

Objectivity was brought in to clinical performance through a novel method of Objective Structured Clinical Examination (OSCE), first described in the year 1975 [6]. Dental graduates were performing clinical skills directly on patients. It has become difficult to get required patients for all the students whose admission strength increased drastically. Evaluators of medical education found OSCE as a gold standard of clinical examination and dentistry followed suit [7, 8]. Students also have endorsed the OSCE [9].

Computer based assessment systems have been tried recently for the classrooms and for self-assessment. They are considered to enhance the learning opportunities.

8.4 Dynamics of Assessment

Assessment is a process that is perceived differently by students, teachers, policymakers and members of the society. From the student's point of view, it is the final destination of a training programme which brands the student as a professional. The teacher or trainer will be interested to know whether the student has learned what is required to practise in society. Both the student and the teacher get feedback. Usually, the students will not pay much attention to the feedback because objective feedback will reveal both strengths and weaknesses. For the teacher it provides an avenue for introspection on the effectiveness of the training programme. The policymakers can get solid information on the programme and get a chance to introduce future modifications. Society is interested in the standard of the health provider so that each one can seek service confidently because the professional is properly assessed. The assessment process got initiated in dental education as a measurement, like knowledge-based and clinical examinations. This was followed by workplace-based assessment. The recent system introduced is the programmatic assessment, where multiple sources of data are collected and collated. The feedback component given is very strong to all the stakeholders, viz. students, teachers, patients, institutions, policymakers and the general public.

8.5 Formative and Summative Assessment

Formative assessment is done to give a feedback to the student on the performance, and it is undertaken periodically to help the student make efforts to improve. This also gives valid feedback to the teachers on their effectiveness. The institution will also get a feedback on the conduct of the programme. In other words, formative assessment shapes student learning and informs the instructor's practice.

Summative assessment is done at the end of the programme to find out whether the candidate is competent enough to be certified. Pass or fail status and ranking are determined through the summative assessment.

8.6 Essential Characteristics or Attributes Required for Assessment

In the earlier days, relevance, validity, reliability, objectivity and feasibility were listed as the essential characteristics of good assessment. But in the present century, the nomenclature has been modified along with the order as follows: Validity, Reliability, Feasibility, and Acceptability and Educational impact.

8.6.1 Validity

The process of assessment should measure the predetermined objectives or the outcome and assess whether the candidate has acquired the knowledge, skills and attitude essential for the practising dentist. A question framed for the written examination, an experiment or clinical step the student is asked to perform and the questions asked in the viva voce should elicit the required outcome. For that, the assessment method and tools should be appropriate. The analogy is that with a measuring tape, we cannot determine the weight of an object. If a weighing balance is given, the weight can be determined. In simplistic terms, this is what is meant by the term validity [10].

Traditionally validity is subdivided into content validity, criterion validity and construct validity. In content validity, the assessment should have adequate coverage of the curriculum encompassing the competencies which are essential for the dentist. Construct validity refers to the construction of an assessment method. If the question has a long-winded phraseology, the doubt raised is whether the intention is to test the subject matter or the ability to comprehend a passage. The questions should be framed carefully so that the intended outcome will be revealed and have sufficient distinctive power. Criterion related validity—a candidate who has a dental degree when appears for the NEET PG exam, which is conducted with the same curricular coverage, may not always qualify. The reason is that, assessment conducted by the University does not reflect the future potential of the candidate. As far as possible this disparity has to be minimised or eliminated from our assessment system.

In modern times, validity is not directly related to the test or questions itself. Usually, people ask whether the test is valid or not. A test may appear valid, but the response or the scores it generates in the group of students selected for the test will help us infer the validity. Suppose we frame a question on the indications of dental implant treatment and administer it to a class of third-year BDS and to second-year MDS students, the scores obtained will be of different patterns and from that we will get an inference whether the assessment is suitable for that set of students or not. All tools are valid or invalid to some extent. A real branding is possible by a careful interpretation of the results. Adequate evidence should be collected to find out whether the assessment has evidence of content, construct and criterion validity. However, it is true that a consensus in the understanding of the term validity cannot be reached easily by the research workers and to some extent by the teachers. That is the reason why the explanations still continue causing at least a minor addition to the existing quantum of confusion [11].

8.6.2 Reliability

The word meaning of 'reliable' is generally twofold: (1) dependable and (2) giving the same results on successive trials. When a written examination is conducted at two different occasions, if the same results or scores are obtained, the assessment is considered reliable. One factor to be considered is that between the tests, there must be considerable time interval; otherwise, the memory factor can cause some bias. Reliability of essay questions is doubtful because on most of the occasions, the scores markedly vary. Modified essay questions and objective-type questions normally have better reliability. The conventional clinical examination of dentistry, involves a patient on him/her the student is expected to demonstrate a clinical step. The competency tested poses limitations because every student will not get a patient with similar features. Hence, objective structured clinical examination (OSCE) was introduced. OSCE has the advantage of many stations where multiple competencies can be assessed. In viva voce, the conventional method is to ask questions directly to the candidate by two or four examiners. Individual bias of examiners, usually mars the reliability of viva voce. Most of the time the scores are dependent on the examiner. Structured viva seems to avoid this bias element in which the candidate is given the option to select a card from a set and that contains eight to ten questions with different difficulty levels (*Bloom's Taxonomy*). It noticeably improves the reliability of viva voce. For BDS examinations, this will bring in a higher order of objectivity. In another method, the questions will be asked by one examiner and the scoring is done by the other. In fact, both the examiner and the examinee will be subjected to assessment; examinee directly and examiner indirectly by the co-examiner.

Checking inter examiner variability in scoring will give an insight into the reliability of assessment. In postgraduate examinations, the theory paper is evaluated by four examiners and hence the reliability profile is very high. The scores are usually averaged. In BDS examinations, the papers are valued by two examiners and if the variation in score is beyond a particular percentage (5 or 10), then the paper is subjected to a third evaluation. This is also a fair method of ensuring reliability of assessment [12]. Reliability can also be tested by preparing two sets of equivalent questions on the same subject matter and assigned randomly amongst the students. The scores can be compared using statistical methods and the reliability can be assessed [13, 14].

8.6.3 Feasibility

Feasibility, practicability and workability have more or less similar meanings. Will a candidate be able to write an answer completely within the stipulated time? Dental clinical examinations are conducted on patients and is it possible to get similar patients for all the candidates? Can we assess professionalism and factors related to affective domain effectively during the assessment sessions?

These are some of the factors faced by the teachers of dentistry. If the questions are framed correctly and the number of items in MCQ-based assessment is properly selected, the feasibility can be improved. The content fit for an essay should not be pushed into the framework of a short answer question. A candidate will find it difficult to include all the contents for 'RRR' in a short answer of 300 words. OSCE to a great extent has solved the problem of getting too many patients with similar features. Professionalism is assessed by newly introduced P-Mex-like systems and newer methods are being researched. In P-Mex, specially designed questionnaire is used so that evaluators can assess the professional attitude of the student [15].

8.6.4 Acceptability

In the assessment process of dentistry, acceptability is a matter of concern for both the students who participate in it and the patients who are subjected to treatment as part of the clinical examination. It should also be acceptable to the teachers who have the role of evaluators and can critically evaluate the validity, reliability and feasibility. Students' acceptability is predominantly related to the fairness factor. Computer-assisted assessments will receive more acceptability if adequate precautions are enforced to prevent cheating. The patient's concern will be with the quality of treatment provided to them. The institutional authorities and the teachers will be more concerned with the addition of infrastructure like computer-integrated labs. When policymakers decide on thc assessment, its feasibility to implement has to be considered and it is no less important than other factors [16, 17].

8.6.5 Educational Impact

Assessment will provide an insight into the student's level of understanding of the subject and the student's strengths and weaknesses. With assessment, the majority of the students will be encouraged to advance further in the learning process and develop a love for learning. They will improve in critical thinking and creativity. It empowers the students to gain life skills, seize opportunities and tackle challenges at professional and personal levels. The society is benefitted by the assessment which ensures the quality of the dental professional who is going to give excellent service. The accuracy or fairness of assessment is important to the student because his future depends on it exclusively. The educational career of the student may be shattered by a wrong decision. Assessment informs the institution and the policymakers whether the career requirements could be satisfactorily completed and suggests dynamic updates in the curriculum [18].

8.7 Programmatic Assessment

The conventional assessment system followed in dental education consists of a written examination, clinical examination and a viva voce conducted at the end of the course period. If the candidate performs well in the clinical examination, the other two components were given less emphasis because all the evaluations were done on the days of the 'examination'. Later, the system of assessing theory papers independently by a separate set of examiners was introduced, to make the process more objective and avoid the 'halo effect'. However, the performance of the candidate during the course period and the pattern of progress during the course period did not have a role in deciding the final assessment. This weakness was identified by van der Vleuten and Schuwirth, the proponents of programmatic assessment [19]. Miller in the earlier days stated that 'assessment drives learning'. Ben David has elaborated the view by stating that 'Assessment expands professional horizons.' [20, 21]. Assessment has to provide an environment conducive to learning and that is an important conceptual change.

Programmatic assessment is a characteristic model of assessment where a decision is taken from information received from multiple sources (known as data points) including the feedback provided. From the multiple data points obtained, crucial decisions can be taken on promotion to the next year of the course and awarding the degree. It also favours of student learning. In 2020, an expert group of members assembled at Ottawa and arrived at a consensus on the principles of programmatic assessment. They are as follows:

1. Every form of assessment used is considered as a data point.
2. Each data point should provide learning by way of feedback to the learner.
3. Pass or fail decision is not taken on the basis of a single data point.
4. The method of assessment chosen should be justifiable on the educational grounds.
5. Multiple methods should be used for assessment.
6. Formative and summative assessments are not made independent but form one continuous process.
7. Decision-making on learner progress is related proportionately to the assessment activities.
8. Information obtained from assessment is interrelated (triangulated) as part of a predetermined framework.
9. High-stakes decisions like promotion and awarding degrees are taken with transparency in a credible manner.
10. Learner progress is subjected to intermediate review involving the learner.
11. Students and faculty should meet to discuss and students are encouraged to do self-analysis of the assessment data.
12. Programmatic assessment ensures a gradual increase of the learner's agency (feeling of having control over one's actions and the consequences produced) and accountability.

8.8 Assessment Tools in the World of Competency-Based Education

The tools are categorised based on *Miller's Pyramid* and the designated levels such as knows, knows how, shows how and does.

8.8.1 Knows

Oral examination, reports prepared by the learner and context-free MCQs are used to test factual recognition.

8.8.2 Knows How

Essays, case-based MCQs and triple jump* are used for assessing the ability to apply the knowledge in the clinical context.

8.8.3 Shows How

OSCE, lab-based practical, simulations and standardised patients are used in a controlled situation.

8.8.4 Does

360^0 assessments, test for clinical competency, direct observation of the candidate's performance, portfolios, video recording, follow-up assessment and clinical triple jump are used to assess the overall performance.

*Triple jump exercise is a three-stage assessment:

1. Student interviews the patient and conducts examination (first jump).
2. Prepares an assessment of the patient and a treatment plan with justified rationale (second jump).
3. Student explains the assessment and treatment plan and answers the questions of the faculty (third jump) [22].

The principles or attributes of good assessment have undergone dynamic changes in understanding and the nomenclature has been subjected to modifications during the last two decades. Presently accepted attributes are as follows:

1. Validity or coherence.
2. Reproducibility or consistency or reliability.
3. Equivalence.
4. Feasibility.
5. Educational impact or effect.
6. Catalytic effect (assessment enhances the educational process).
7. Acceptability [23–25].

In the course of revision, two attributes have been eliminated, viz. relevance and objectivity. These two factors are, in fact, included in the validity, which is upgraded in the hierarchy to the first position. Assessment in the recent times has undergone multidimensional changes which has altered the meaning from a pass/fail tool to a learning support system. The future dentist coming out of our institutions will definitely be competent in the desired skills capable of thinking and interested in lifelong learning.

8.9 Towards Mastery

To become an expert in any profession, it requires 10 years of intense practice. Malcom Gladwell in his bestselling book, '*Outliers: The Story of Success*' stated that 'you need 10,000 hours of deliberate practice to achieve mastery in a particular skill' [26].

Mastery development happens in five stages:

1. Novice.
2. Beginner.
3. Competent.
4. Proficient.
5. Mastery or expertise.

Novice A student who has just joined a training programme is the novice and has no previous experience. A Novice cannot take decisions independently and is always dependent on the faculty. They meticulously follow the rules of the institution or the teacher. In the first 2 years of any professional course, students remain as novices.

Beginner Candidates in the third and fourth year and during the internship are considered as the beginners. Dependency on the teacher in decision-making continues and when a familiar situation arises, they may perform with confidence. But in different contexts, they may find it difficult to perform. Beginners are comparatively faster and more accurate than novices in their skills and decisions.

Competent In this stage, a professional gains capability to do practise independently. They can manage most of the clinical situations in a professional manner since they have acquired the skills and internalised the standards of performance.

Proficiency In this stage, the professional can gauge the scope and limitations of his practising field. He ventures into experimenting with the recent developments of the profession and can adapt his skills to face challenging situations.

Mastery or Expertise After many years of practice, a professional gains mastery. He will start contributing towards the profession by way of new knowledge and skills and will share these with others through scientific articles and by conducting training programmes. A professional passes through many phases of a reinvention process to reach the mastery stage. This categorisation of professional expertise was given by Chambers D W and it can be considered as the initiating attempt towards competency-based education [27, 28].

> Good teaching is more a giving of right questions
> than a giving of right answers
> -Josef Albers
> German-American artist and educator

References

1. Broadfoot P, Black P. Redefining assessment? The first ten years of assessment in education. Assess Educ Prin Policy Pract. 2004;11(1):7–26. https://doi.org/10.1080/0969594042000208976.
2. Marzano RJ. Class room assessment and grading that work. Rediff Books; 2006.
3. Earl L. Assessment as learning: using classroom assessment to maximise student learning. Thousand Oaks: Corwin Press; 2003.
4. https://learnercentered.org/author/bryanna-hanson/
5. https://getscorpion.caveon.com/the-future-of-multiple-choice/
6. Harden R, Stevenson M, Downie W, Wilson G. Assessment of clinical competence using objective structured examination. Br Med J. 1975;1:447–51. [CrossRef] [PubMed]
7. Manogue M, Brown G. Developing and implementing an OSCE in dentistry. Eur J Dent Educ. 1998;2:51–7. [CrossRef] [PubMed]
8. Mossey P, Newton J, Stirrups D. Scope of the OSCE in the assessment of clinical skills in dentistry. Br Dent J. 2001;190:323–6. [CrossRef] [PubMed]
9. Puryer J. Dental undergraduate views of objective structured clinical examinations (OSCEs): a literature review. Dent J. 2016;4:6. https://doi.org/10.3390/dj4010006.
10. Vleuten S. Assessment of professional competence from methods to programs. Med Educ. 39:309–17.
11. Royal KD. Four tenets of modern validity theory for medical education assessment and evaluation. Adv Med Educ Pract. 2017;8:567–70.
12. Cohen J. A coefficient of agreement for nominal scales. Educ Psychol Meas. 1960;20:37–46.
13. DeVellis RF. Scale development: theory and applications. Thousand Oaks: SAGE; 2016.
14. Nu MN, Htay MG, Kamath AKM, Sugathan S, Luyee EO, Sahoo S. Overview of reliability and validity of assessments in medical education. Int J Transform Health Prof Educ. 2023;1:19–26.
15. Cruess R, McIlroy JH, Cruess S, Ginsburg S, Steinert Y. The professionalism mini-evaluation exercise: a preliminary investigation. Acad Med. 2006;81:574–8.
16. Sekhon, et al. Development of a theory-informed questionnaire to assess the acceptability of healthcare interventions. BMC Health Serv Res. 2022;22:279.
17. Escudier MP, Tricio JA, Odell EW. Student acceptability of high-stakes e-assessment in dental education: using privacy screen filters to control cheating. J Dent Educ. 2014;78(4):558–66.
18. https://www.watermarkinsights.com/resources/blog/educational-impact#
19. Van Der Vleuten C, Schuwirth L, Driessen E, Dijkstra J, Tigelaar D, Baartman L, Van Tartwijk J. A model for programmatic assessment fit for purpose. Med Teach. 2012;34(3):205–14.

20. Miller G. The assessment of clinical skills/competence/performance. Acad Med. 1990;65(9):S63–7.
21. Ben-David MF. The role of assessment in expanding professional horizons. Med Teach. 2000;22(5):472–7.
22. Albino JEN, Young SK, Neumann LM, Kramer GA, Andrieu SC, Henson L, Horn B, Hendricson WD. Assessing dental students' competence: best practice recommendations in the performance assessment literature and investigation of current practices in predoctoral dental education. J Dent Educ. 2008;72:1405–35.
23. Norcini J, Anderson MB, Bollela V, Burch V, Costa MG, Duvivier R. 2018 Consensus frame work for good assessment. Med Teach. 2018;40:1102–9.
24. Ananthakrishnan N, et al., editors. Medical education principles and practice. 2nd ed. Pondicherry: National Teacher Training Centre, JIPMER; 2000.
25. Singh T, et al. Principles of assessment in medical education. 2nd ed. New Delhi: Jaypee Brothers Medical Publishers; 2024.
26. Gladwell M. Outliers-the story of success. Penguin Books; 2009.
27. Chambers DW. Competency-based dental education in context. Eur J Dent Educ. 1998;2(1):8–13.
28. Koshy E, Nair C, Dathan P, et al. Competency based dental education—a narrative review. Acta Sci Dent Sci. 2024;8(8):74–83.

9 Setting a Reliable and Valid Question Paper

Elbe Peter

Understanding a question is half an answer
Socrates

9.1 Introduction

The most traditional and universally accepted method of assessment across any discipline of learning is the written examination with the help of a question paper (QP). Dental science is no exception. Here, the QP serves as the tool to measure how much a student has learnt. Any teacher would have set numerous question papers in their teaching career, with or without fully understanding the essential principles. A QP set without adhering to the essential principles becomes a poor instrument of measurement. The primary goal of any good educator is to impart knowledge, skills, and values to the students. It is the duty of the educator to ensure that students not only acquire these competencies but can also apply them effectively in unsupervised environments [1]. In dentistry it is the duty of a dental teacher to ensure that the student is competent and safe to practice dentistry in the public domain. Assessment is the most accepted means to ensure learning. Different domains of learning require different assessment methods. The cognitive domain is primarily assessed through written tests using a well-prepared, reliable, and valid question paper. This chapter focuses on setting a reliable and valid question paper, including the preparation of a blueprint.

E. Peter (✉)
Government Dental College, Thrissur, Kerala, India

Kerala University of Health Sciences, Thrissur, Kerala, India
e-mail: dean.dental@kuhs.ac.in

R. M. Baiju, S. Thomas (eds.), *The Dental Teacher*,
https://doi.org/10.1007/978-3-032-07551-2_9

- QP is a tool of measurement, it should be set carefully for being a valid measure
- It primarily measures the cognitive domain of learning

9.2 Need for a Question Paper

A systematically prepared question paper for a written examination can be analogously compared to a reliable and valid questionnaire used for data collection in research. It should be well-balanced in terms of its content aligning with the syllabus, the knowledge being assessed and its domain levels, and the types of questions. As mentioned earlier, a QP primarily assesses the cognitive domain of the subject and serves as the instrument for its measurement. It serves as a means of communication between the candidate and the educator. Hence, it should possess certain qualities and meet specific standards [1], which will be discussed further in this chapter.

9.3 Qualities of a Good Question Paper

- Validity
- Reliability
- Relevance
- Comprehensive syllabus coverage
- Well-framed—considering time-to-complete factor
- Clear and unambiguous
- Discriminative between high and low achievers

Validity and reliability are two inherent properties that must be possessed by any measuring instrument, providing insight into how effectively the method measures the intended criteria. Validity refers to the accuracy of a measure (i.e. whether the results truly represent what they are supposed to measure). Reliability refers to the consistency of a measure (i.e. whether the results can be reproduced under similar conditions). The difference is depicted in Fig. 9.1.

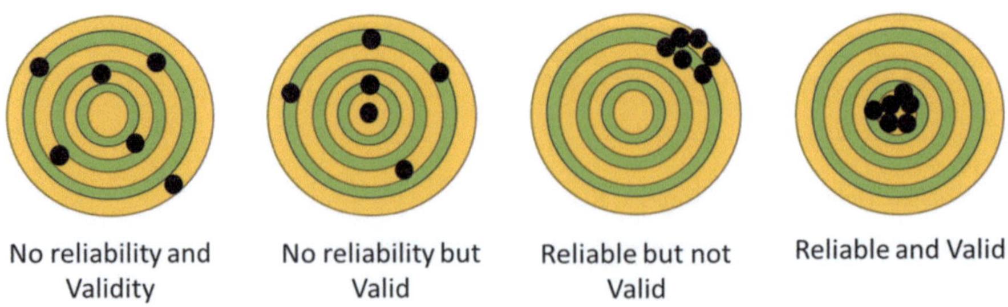

Fig. 9.1 Difference between reliability and validity

Validity is influenced by a host of factors, including the qualities listed above. It measures the 'truthfulness' of a question paper, i.e. whether it measures what a test is intended to measure. Using a poorly valid instrument can lead to incorrect interpretations. For example, using an underrepresented question paper covering only a part of a particular syllabus can yield erroneous conclusions about a student's learning. The types of validity applicable to a question paper include face validity, content validity, criterion validity and convergent validity.

Face validity refers to the test takers' response or overall perception of the question paper, often expressed as 'easy', 'difficult', or a response in between. Content validity, on the other hand, should be ensured by experts in the field. It ensures that the question paper aligns with the syllabus and adheres to criteria such as the percentage of questions from specific areas, levels of difficulty, adequate representation of content areas, etc. It should not be erroneously concluded that when an expert in the field rates the QP as easy, it need not be so because the test takers are novices and not experts. This factor should be kept in mind when setting the QP. Content validity, Criterion validity, and Convergent validity collectively form what is known as Construct validity or Statistical validity. These estimates are specifically assessed in questionnaires used in research to ensure the psychometric properties of the instrument and, in turn, to ensure the validity of the study. However, in the strict sense, these are not so well measured in a question paper, though they are important. Convergent validity can be assumed when another form of test measuring a similar construct produces similar results. Conversely, differing results indicate divergent validity.

The reliability of a question paper is essential because the aim of an assessor is to test the knowledge domains of the test taker consistently, however, it may not be feasible to repeat the test. Hence, the test prepared, i.e. the question paper should possess all features that ensure reliability. Adhering to the other qualities of a question paper inherently ensures reliability. In addition, the length of the question paper also influences reliability; a greater number of questions ensure better reliability. However, for most institutions and universities, the number of questions in a question paper is fixed. Within these limits, careful structuring of questions, especially essay-type questions, contributes to objectivity and, in turn, reliability. Additionally, using unambiguous terms in the stem of the questions ensures reliability. From a statistical point of view, a shorter retest interval improves reliability.

Relevance of the questions in a question paper is the basic principle that ensures the validity of the question paper. Irrelevant questions or those from trivial areas of the syllabus undermine the validity of the test. On the other hand, coverage of a wide range of topics ensures the representativeness of the test. However, as most institutions and universities have a fixed number of questions in a question paper, referring to a well-prepared blueprint whilst setting can ensure adequate coverage.

Well-framed questions ensure clarity and eliminate ambiguity for the students. The correct use of syntax, question wording, punctuation and other details is important for clear understanding and contributes to both the reliability and validity of the question paper. The time allotted to complete the paper is another crucial factor to be kept in mind whilst setting a question paper. It is important to keep in mind that it is the students, not the teachers, who are taking the test. What may seem easy for teachers may not be the same for students. They should also get adequate time to review their answers prior to submission.

The recent trend of online examinations, where the system automatically submits the paper at the end of the stipulated time, necessitates provisions for revisiting previously answered or flagged questions. This aspect should be considered when addressing the time-to-complete factor in question paper setting. A well-prepared question paper should be discriminative in nature, i.e. it should be able to differentiate between high achievers and low achievers. Referring to institutional norms regarding the QP pattern is important prior to setting a question paper. On an average, 60%–70% questions should be from the must-to-know areas, 20%–30% from good-to-know areas of the syllabus, and 10% from desirable-to-know areas. This pattern ensures the discriminative power of the question paper.

- Validity setting ensures the candidate's knowledge in the content area.
- Reliability ensures that the candidate's knowledge is consistent.
- Avoid ambiguous terms in the QP and questions of trivial nature.
- Time-to-complete factor and discriminative power between high and low achievers should be kept in mind.

9.4 Steps in Question Paper Designing and Blueprinting

1. Deciding on the design
2. Preparing the blueprint
3. Preparing a model QP (including the answer key)
4. Preparing the marking scheme
5. Refining the QP
6. Editing
7. Review

9.4.1 Design of a Question Paper

Design of a question paper is largely a policy matter decided by the apex body or the University [1]. It is based on the curriculum, syllabus, and required competencies. The number and types of questions, marking schemes, duration of the question paper, and sections to be included in the paper are thus pre-decided by the University or apex body. The design of the QP for a particular course is an end product of numerous modifications and refinements that have happened in the subject over many years. Once the apex body overseeing the assessment process approves a design, it should be adhered to by the QP setters. The duration of the test for a particular course, number of items in the QP, types of items, its format, etc. are pre-decided and communicated to the QP setters (Table 9.1).

Table 9.1 List of items communicated to the setter prior to setting of a question paper

1	Syllabus of the course
2	Instructions regarding the setting of the question paper
3	Sample question paper
4	Writing/printing paper with university stamp/seal (optional)
5	Postal cover/seal for returning (optional)
6	Remuneration details and bills

9.4.2 Preparing the Question Paper (QP) Blueprint

Blueprinting refers to the framework of the question paper. It is usually decided by the university and provided to teachers, or it may be left to teachers to prepare a blueprint based on the syllabus. The topics are categorised according to the course content and their weightage. In the disease model of healthcare, the impact (I) of a condition (disease) and its frequency (F) can be used as a guide to derive the weightage coefficient. However, this approach may not always be feasible across all specialties of dentistry. A rough outline is presented below:

1. Impact of the condition on oral/general health (I)

   (non-urgent = 1, urgent = 2, very urgent = 3)

2. Frequency of the condition (F)

   (rare = 1, relatively common = 2, very common = 3)

Weightage coefficient of a topic is calculated by multiplying the impact score (I) by the frequency score (F), and then dividing the result by the total sum (T) of all I × F scores across the syllabus.

$$\text{Weightage coefficient} = \mathrm{I} \times \mathrm{F} / \mathrm{T}, \mathrm{T} = \Sigma(\mathrm{I} \times \mathrm{F})(\text{total of } \mathrm{I} \times \mathrm{F} \text{ scores})$$

In dental subjects, it may not always be feasible to precisely calculate the impact score and frequency score for all specialties; many topics extend beyond mere conditions (disease) and their treatments. In such cases, experts can determine the weightage scores based on its relative importance of each topic. The number of items (questions in KUHS QP) is pre-decided: for UG papers, there are 16 in each, and for PG, there are 10 questions in Part 1. In PG Part 2, Papers 1 and 2 contain 7 questions (2 Essays for 25 marks each and 5 short essays for 10 marks each), whilst Paper 3 has 3 essay questions, of which 2 must be answered.

The weightage score (w) multiplied by the total number of questions in the QP will determine the number of questions to be asked from that area and 'w' multiplied by the total marks for the paper will give the percentage of marks to be allotted to that content area.

It can be a laborious task initially to prepare a blue print for a course, but once prepared, the same can be used every year with necessary updation. The time spent in its preparation is worthwhilst for the validity of the assessment. Inputs should be taken from faculty members of all levels in deciding the weightage score and identifying the types of items and test questions for each weightage area.

9.4.3 Preparation of a Model Question Paper (QP) with Answer Key

The next step is to prepare the model question paper QP along with the answer key. The number of answer points to be written and the corresponding marks for each point should be clearly mentioned for descriptive questions. The time-to-complete factor is a very important aspect in any QP designing. The allocated time for each question should be kept in mind and final revision time is also important. Preparation of a model QP and answer key will help to avoid overlooking this important concept.

9.4.4 Marking Scheme

The marking scheme assigns proportions of marks to different parts of the answer. Marking schemes can be categorised as either analytical or global:

- ***Analytical marking scheme***: This is the most widely adopted approach across all dental specialties for both undergraduate (UG) and postgraduate (PG) assessments. In this scheme, questions are properly structured, with appropriate question verbs aligned with the desired learning level. Marks are allocated for each subdivision of the answer. This approach is expected to be more objective and tends to demonstrate good inter-assessor reliability.
- ***Global marking scheme***: Typically used for MDS Paper 3 long essay-type questions. In this case, questions are usually unstructured and scoring can vary significantly between evaluators. Consequently, this scheme is more subjective and may lead to higher variability in marks awarded.

9.4.5 Refining of the Question Paper (QP)

The set model paper should be critically assessed and refined at this stage. The QP setter now should consider certain important points whilst refining, like the learning outcome and objectives of the topic, clarity of the questions, language used, marking scheme, difficulty level and time to complete the QP. The QP should be relevant to the course specific outcome envisaged. Questions from unimportant and trivial areas should be avoided. The length of the QP should be such that it should be reasonably feasible for an average student to write and review their answers before submission. Mark allotment should be proportional to the length of the answer and difficulty level. Uniform coverage of the entire syllabus should be ensured. Instructions provided and language used in the QP should be clear and understandable to an average student taking the test. Grammatical errors, typos etc. should be avoided as it can alter the meaning and create confusions. Following checklist (Table 9.2) can help the QP setter to prevent overlooking any aspect whilst refining the question paper.

Table 9.2 Check list to be considered whilst refining a QP

1	Does the question test an important learning outcome?
2	Is it based on a predetermined objective?
3	Are the instructions given clearly?
4	Is the language (especially action verbs) unambiguous?
5	Is the time-to-complete factor considered or not (length of the written answer)?
6	Has the marking scheme and subdivisions provided?
7	Is the difficulty level appropriate for the test takers?

Adapted and modified from Reddy K R

9.4.6 Editing

Editing of the QP should take care of the grouping of the questions according to the objectives, contents, and other relevant factors. Repeat questions from the same content area should be avoided. Proper numbering and instructions for administration should be carefully checked. If the question paper extends to additional pages, it should be mentioned.

9.4.7 Reviewing

Final step is to review the prepared QP. Here, the points considered above are thoroughly reviewed before dispatching the question paper. Following points should be considered whilst reviewing the QP.

- Fair coverage of the syllabus
- Weightage to appropriate content areas ensured by following the blueprint
- Level of difficulty (for an average student) factor
- Discriminative power of the QP
- Overlap of questions
- Ambiguous action verbs or terms
- Time-to-complete factor
- Repetition of questions appearing in previous papers avoided as much as possible
- Whether the QP is of comparable standard with that of previous years' QP
- Is the QP testing the abilities prescribed in the regulations or syllabus
- Typos and grammatical errors should be checked

The eighth or final step is to ensure the confidentiality of the set QP. The draft papers should be destroyed and final QP should be sealed properly and send to the university following the instructions. If asked for soft copy or via mail, necessary password protection of the file should be ensured.

- Blueprinting is identification of the weightage coefficient for the content area and helps to decide the number of questions and marks for each domain.
- Proper structuring and clear marking scheme are important
- Refining and editing ensure completeness and correctness of the QP

9.5 Question Paper Scrutiny

Universities typically adopt a policy where question paper setters are handpicked from other institutions or universities and invited to prepare a few sets of question papers. These papers are then scrutinised by qualified and expert faculty members of the parent university, which is going to use these QPs. This process of scrutiny of the question paper is the final opportunity for making corrections and to ensure alignment with the scheme followed in that institution. Hence, the scrutiny of the question paper is another important task that has to be done carefully, adhering to the principles enlisted above, by competent faculty members. It is a highly confidential process and any changes or modifications made should be substantiated with a reason.

9.6 Types of Questions in a Question Paper (QP)

The questions or items in a question paper are the most important factors. These items are designed to measure the knowledge of the students. In a way, it is similar to the items in a psychometric questionnaire. The basic principles to be followed when designing the questions are that they should be simple to understand, unambiguous, definite, clear, and answerable. Most universities prefer a mix of questions, including essay questions, modified essay questions, short answer questions, brief notes, or multiple-choice questions.

Essay & short answer questions are among the most commonly used methods for summative assessment in BDS/MDS courses. They are primarily used to assess the cognitive domains of learning. An essay is a piece of writing that methodically analyses and evaluates a topic or issue [2]. Improper question formulation often compromises the validity and reliability of the examination and leads to various hassles for both students and examiners. Modified Essay Questions, on the other hand, are mostly applied in clinical medical or dental sciences where a description of a condition or problem is presented, followed by related questions. Short Answer Questions (SAQs) are usually the most frequent and preferred type of questions in a standard dental QP, assessing cognitive knowledge, especially in the lower domains. In contrast, Multiple Choice Questions (MCQs) are often asked in screening and pre-test questionnaires. Certain universities include MCQs in both formative and summative assessments as well. Well-constructed MCQs can assess learning in multiple domains, but primarily focus on the cognitive domain, and can do so at various levels.

Each type of question has its own advantages and disadvantages, which are described briefly below.

- Essay Questions
- Modified Essay Questions
- Short Answer Questions
- Brief Answer Questions
- Multiple Choice Questions

9.7 Essay Questions (EQs)

Essay-type questions are open-ended type questions where the test taker should construct a response in the form of sentences, paragraphs etc. Here, students should compose their own answer rather than selecting a response from the given options [3]. They are inevitable in dental assessments because they help measure complex learning outcomes like higher order cognitive skills such as the ability to reason, create, analyse, synthesise, and evaluate. They provide a comprehensive evaluation of the student's knowledge and encourage them to be original and flexible in their responses. John M. Stalnkar defined essay type questions are the 'test items which require a response composed by the examinee, usually in the form of one or more sentences of a nature that no single response or pattern of response can be listed as correct, and the accuracy and quality of which can be judged subjectively only by one skilled or informed in the subject' [4]. According to Robert L. E. and David A. F., an essay type test presents tasks that require extended written responses from the person being tested [5]. The main purpose of an essay question is to assess the student's understanding of the subject matter and their ability to reason with the knowledge of the subject.

Types of Essays/Constructed Response Questions

1. Open-ended essays
2. Closed ended essays

Or

1. Long answer/extended response essay
2. Short answer/restricted response essay

Restricted Response (Closed Ended/Structured) Essays: The students' response is restricted.

For example, *classify red and white lesions in the oral cavity. Write in detail the clinical manifestations, laboratory investigations and management of oral leukoplakia. (3 + 3 + 2 + 2)*

- Places a strict limit in the response
- The question is specific.
- Adjectives like 'List', 'Define', Enumerate, Outline, etc. are used.
- It is more structured with exact mark distribution.
- Measures specific learning outcome
- Ease of valuing the answer script

Extended Response (Open Ended/Unstructured) Essays: The students' response is unrestricted here.

For example, *discuss various plaque control methods—10 marks*

- Learning outcome of higher cognitive levels is assessed.
- Creative ability, analysis, synthesis etc. are measured.
- Scoring is unreliable and difficult.

9.7.1 Basic Response Format for an Essay

- A basic essay response consists of three main parts: introduction, body and conclusion.
- Introduction guides to the paper by grabbing attention and introducing the topic—can include definitions or general concepts or epidemiological facts on the topic.
- The body can begin with a statement regarding the main idea followed by elaboration of main points in further paragraphs.
- The body paragraphs should be set in the order of ideas and should have a smooth transition from one to the next. Bullet points can be added to convey more information. Additionally neat and labelled diagrams can be drawn for better explaining.
- The conclusion brings together all the major points of the essay and should leave the readers with a final thought and sense of closure.
- If any outside information or research paper is referred to, credits should be given to the source.

9.7.2 Essay Questions: Strengths

1. Best tool to assess factual knowledge—knowledge gained from multiple sources
2. The student's ability to answer the question (expressing ideas, organizing) can be assessed.
3. Assess complex learning outcomes—abilities to select, organise, integrate, relate, and evaluate ideas.
4. Essays encourage students to develop more desirable study habits because they encourage the production of written language and the expression of thought.
5. They are relatively easy to construct and do not take much time to set. Hence, they have practicability as an advantage to them.

6. Encourage creativity.
7. Non-content attributes such as basic language, handwriting, and time management can also be assessed.

9.7.3 Essay Questions: Limitations for Evaluators

1. Limited validity—large size limits the number of test items. Therefore, it will assess only very few areas of the curriculum. Hence, essay question may cause under-sampling/oversampling of the content domain.
2. Poor reliability—unlikely that the students will perform exactly the same way as on the previous occasion.
3. Highly subjective—the unlimited scope of the essay leaves considerable room for subjective judgement. Superfluous factors such as bad handwriting & poor spelling/grammar may undermine an otherwise good answer. On the other hand, a student may bluff his way to better marks through smart writing.
4. No single answer can be considered correct or perfect
5. Takes long time to score
6. The essay questions are often framed in a non-descript phrases, giving students no idea about the scope of the answer expected.
7. The wording of an essay question is critical to ensure what is asked aligns with what is understood.

9.7.4 Common Misconceptions Regarding Essay Questions

- Assess higher-order or critical thinking skills regardless of how they are written.
- Essay questions are easy to construct.
- The use of essay questions eliminates the problem of guessing.
- Essay questions benefit all students by placing emphasis on the importance of written communication skills.
- Essay questions encourage students to prepare more thoroughly.

9.7.5 How to Effectively Construct a Standard Essay Question?

- Clearly define the intended learning outcome to be assessed by the item
- Clearly define the task. Delimit the scope of the task. Clearly develop the problem/problem situation.
- Present a reasonable task to students in the form of a statement or question
- State the criteria for grading by clearly specifying the mark allotment and writing a model answer.
- Better to avoid the use of optional questions
- Improve the essay question through preview and peer review

- Make problem-based structured essay questions with checklists. The wording of the question should limit the scope of the content and direct the student to a precise and specific response. This will improve the reliability of the test.
- Carefully structure the parts of the question. The question must be framed in a manner that student can answer subsequent parts even if he/she does not know one part of the answer.

9.7.6 Measures to Overcome the Disadvantages of Essays

1. Use a detailed test blue print and test specification. This can prevent undersampling or biased sampling.
2. Use of structured or modified essay questions limits the content and thus the item is made more objective.
3. The wording of an essay question is critical- to ensure what is asked aligns with what is understood.
4. It is desirable to create a question bank at the department level and use it during internal assessments so that the construction of essay questions is consistently improved.
5. Evaluation by independent experts regarding the cognitive levels can improve validity.
6. Evaluation bias due to inherent subjectivity can be reduced by using two or more evaluators who are well trained and with the use of model answers.
7. Use of formal model answer: These can show the students the standards you expect from them & also help you in awarding marks.

9.8 Modified Essay Questions (MEQ)

Modified essay questions (MEQ) are one method to overcome the disadvantages of open-ended/unstructured essay questions. They are usually presented as short clinical scenarios followed by a series of questions with a structured format for scoring. They mainly assess the student's factual recall but can also assess cognitive skills, such as organisation of knowledge, reasoning, and problem solving. It can also address the writing skills and even ethical, social and moral issues, and attitudes. MEQs are more flexible and their value is somewhere between essay type questions and SAQ's. They should be carefully constructed with provision of model answers and training to avoid inter-rater variability. One example for MEQ can be as follows:

- An apprehensive mother brings her 12-year-old daughter to the dental OPD with a concern about midline diastema between the central incisors. On examination, the patient presented in the mixed dentition stage with permanent canines unerupted. The molar relation is Class I with mild deep bite of 6 mm, over jet of 4 mm. Cephalometric evaluation revealed SNA of 84 degrees, SNB of 82 degrees, and Mandibular plane angle of 26 degrees. OPG revealed the presence of permanent maxillary canines. Outline your diagnosis, differential diagnosis, and mode of management. Give a brief note on causes of midline diastema and various schools of management.

Whilst constructing MEQ, care should be exercised regarding the correctness of the clinical condition described and ensure that no clue to the diagnosis or treatment planning is provided in the subsequent sub-questions.

9.9 Short Answer Questions (SAQs)

They are open-ended questions which require students to create an answer [6]. Though similar to essay questions, the length of the answer is limited.

9.9.1 What Is Assessed by Short Answer Questions?

SAQs are commonly used in examinations to assess the students' basic knowledge and understanding of a topic (lower cognitive levels).

9.9.2 Types of Short Answer Questions

- In general, there are two types of short-answer exam questions: factual (i.e. testing memory work) and interpretive (i.e. testing your ability to apply learnt concepts).
  - **Factual short-answer questions:** The function of factual questions is to describe or define the way things are. They often use the following instruction words: *Define, Give, Identify, List, Name, Outline, Provide, State,* etc.
  - **Interpretive short-answer questions:** Interpretive questions test the ability of the students to apply their knowledge. Interpretive questions often use the following instruction words: Account for…, Comment on..., Compare..., Consider..., Contrast..., Describe..., Discuss..., Distinguish..., Elaborate on.., etc.

9.9.3 Comparison of Long Essay Question with Short Answer Question

Long answer/extended response essay	Short answer question
1. Tests deeper sampling of narrow domain 2. Assesses the cognitive domain. Tests knowledge objectives at higher levels. It assesses complex cognitive skills, including analysis, synthesis, and evaluation. It measures the ability to research a topic, organise, integrate, evaluate ideas, construct and present it in coherent English. It also assesses the student's factual knowledge and recall knowledge 3. There is freedom of response to the question 4. The response contains more than one sentence	1. Tests broader sampling of domain 2. Tests lower domains of learning. It assesses only factual knowledge, recall knowledge, and the ability to apply 3. Boundaries are set on the answer required and on its organisation 4. Students may be required to write a word, phrase/sentence to complete a statement

9.10 Brief Answer Questions (BAQs)

Brief Answer Questions (or Brief Notes) are a format with an even shorter version of Short Answer Questions. Here, the candidates are expected to provide three to four bullet points as answers. This is commonly followed for undergraduate students by the Kerala University of Health Sciences (KUHS). Answers in this format should be of least descriptive type, presenting only the crux of the matter in concise points. Great caution should be exercised when setting this type of question. The question should be highly specific so that the candidate can answer precisely. Vague questions without a proper stem will attract ambiguity, forcing students to write lengthy descriptive responses instead.

Examples of brief answer/note questions

List three advantages of removable orthodontic appliance
Define an index
Write four side effects of metronidazole
Differentiate between growth and development

The advantage of this type of question is its objectivity, which is higher than SAQ, and its ease of evaluation.

9.11 Multiple Choice Questions (MCQs)

It is one of the most frequently and widely used assessment tools in undergraduate and postgraduate medical education. Though it is commonly used in formative assessments and selection (entrance) examinations, its role cannot be neglected in summative examinations as well. The National Dental Commission (NDC) recommends the use of all forms of questions for assessment, including multiple choice questions in summative assessments. However, a thorough understanding of how to set an MCQ is important to prepare effective test questions.

9.11.1 Structure of a MCQ

The main body of the question is the Stem. The response options are the Distractors (wrong answers) and the Key (the right answer). For example:

Pit and fissure sealant application is a form of: **(Stem)**

A. Primary prevention
B. Secondary prevention
C. Tertiary prevention
D. Primordial prevention

A—Key (correct answer) **B, C, D—Distractors**
Some MCQ's may have a task called the Lead-In question

A 32-year-old female patient who underwent an uneventful extraction of 26 in the morning was brought to the OPD in the evening with oozing of blood from the socket. Patient had no remarkable history and vitals are normal.

What will be your first choice of management? **Lead – in**

A. Pressure pack
B. Immediate shifting to a tertiary care centre
C. IV injection of Tranexamic acid
D. Put the patient on anti-hypertensives

9.11.2 Levels of Learning Targeted by MCQs

MCQs can be designed to specifically test student learning at levels such as remembering, understanding and applying [6, 7]. With careful construction, even higher cognitive domains can be tested using MCQ.

9.11.3 Advantages of MCQ Based Assessment

1. Large number of candidates can be assessed in a short time and cost-effective manner.
2. The 'correct' answers are predetermined, and do not involve subjective judgements as required in written examinations.
3. Validity of assessment of cognitive domain can be improved by ensuring coverage of the entire syllabus and preparing questions to assess different levels of knowledge.

4. The lack of dependence on paper-based questions permits substantial flexibility in both the location and the timing of the exam.
5. MCQs can be easily administered either on paper or electronically (Google forms/Moodle).
6. It is easy to electronically vary the order in which questions are presented to the candidates.

9.11.4 Limitations of MCQ Based Assessment

1. Poor validity for assessment of psychomotor/affective domain
2. May be confusing if not prepared properly
3. Multiple-choice assessments are open to abuse through guessing
4. Constructing good test items is challenging and requires significant time and effort

9.11.5 Features of a 'Good' MCQ

1. A good MCQ assesses a clearly identified concept or learning objective.
2. The stem will be derived from a specific item within the curriculum.
3. The question should test concepts of understanding or data evaluation and should avoid simple tasks such as recall or pattern recognition.
4. The stem contains all information that is necessary to answer the question and nothing more.
5. A consistent degree of plausibility in each of the distractors is highly desirable. However, a question where one or two distractors are weaker than the others may not necessarily function as a 'bad' question.
6. The correct/incorrect distractors must be justifiable using an evidence base.
7. The question is positively worded (i.e. does not use EXCEPT, NOT, etc.).
8. Avoidance of concepts such as 'all of the above', 'none of the above', 'answers 2 and 3 only', etc.
9. Each question should be self-contained and not refer directly to another question.
10. It should not be possible to deduce the answer of one question from the information presented in a previous or subsequent question.

9.11.6 Tips for Writing Multiple-Choice Questions

1. Use plausible distractors (wrong-response options)
   - Only list plausible distractors, even if the number of options per question changes
   - Write the options so they are homogeneous in content

- Use answers given in previous open-ended exams to provide realistic distractors

2. Use a Question Format—experts encourage multiple-choice items to be prepared as questions (rather than incomplete statements)
3. Emphasise higher-level thinking—use questions that test higher levels of cognitive domain
4. Keep option lengths similar—avoid making the correct answer noticeably longer or shorter
5. Balance the placement of the correct answer
6. Be grammatically correct—use simple, precise, and unambiguous wording. Students are more likely to select the correct answer by finding the grammatically correct option
7. Avoid clues to the correct answer
8. Use only one correct option (or be sure the best option is clearly the best answer)
9. Do not use MCQ's available from guides/books. Prepare them freshly, providing references from standard textbooks/journals
10. Combine standard MCQ with image-based questions to improve validity

9.11.7 Steps in Writing MCQ'S

Step 1: Choose the learning objectives for which you want to write an MCQ
Step 2: Write your Stem and Lead-in—For MCQs that target learning at the 'remembering' or 'understanding' levels, the stem is often very brief and may not require a lead-in. Use '**WOOF- which one of the following**....' format for lead-in in clinical scenarios/higher order questions
Step 3: Write the correct answer
Step 4: Write the distractors
Step 5: Check for pitfalls
Step 6: Review and edit with a partner

- Essay Questions—tests higher cognitive domains, encourage creativity, assess non-content attributes of writing
- Modified Essay Questions—good choice for problem-solving type questions
- Short Answer Questions—more objective and moderately descriptive
- Brief Answer Questions—answer to-the-point type questions, objective, & specific in nature
- Multiple Choice Questions—most objective type, easy to grade, usually assess lower domains.

9.12 Conclusion

Setting a reliable and valid question paper is not easy, but is an essential job of a teacher. One should devote time and effort to have a meaningful assessment process in place in any dental education scenario. Adhering to the principles highlighted can simplify this task. The following key points can be drawn from the above discussion:

- QP should be valid & reliable.
- It must align with the syllabus and scheme.
- Only standard abbreviations should be used in a question paper (QP).
- The level of difficulty should be average for the majority of the test takers.
- Split-up of marks for structured essays should be clear and based on the quantum of knowledge and difficulty, not the volume of writing.
- Consider including diagrams, problem-solving questions, etc.
- Question paper scrutiny is the last step to rectify errors in question paper setting adopted by the Universities; hence it should be done carefully.

References

1. Reddy KR. Mechanics of question paper setting. J Gandaki Med College-Nepal. 2017;10(2):64–7.
2. Reiner MC, Bothell TW, Sudweeks RR. Preparing effective essay questions. A self-directed workbook for educators. Stillwater: New Forum Press; 2002.
3. Reiner CM, Bothell TW, Sudweeks RR, Wood B. Preparing effective essay questions—a self-directed workbook for educators. New Forums Press; 2002.
4. Stalnaker JM. The essay type of examination. In: Lindquist EF, editor. Educational measurement. Menasha: George Banta; 1951. p. 495–530.
5. Ebel RL, Frisbie DA. Essentials of educational measurement. 5th ed. Englewood Cliffs: Prentice Hall; 1991.
6. Kar SS, Lakshminarayanan S, Mahalakshmy T. Basic principles of constructing multiple choice questions. Indian J Community Family Med. 2015;1(2):65–9.
7. Haladyna TM, Downing SM, Rodriguez MC. A review of multiple-choice item-writing guidelines for classroom assessment. Appl Meas Educ. 2002;15(3):309–34.

Conducting an Oral Examination

10

A. Devadathan and P. R. Rekha

10.1 Introduction

The success of any educational system depends on proper assessment. In medical education, the evaluations of students are done by theory examinations, practical examinations and oral examinations or viva voce. The evaluation of the cognitive domain is the main focus of the theory examination. Here, primary consideration is given to student's knowledge, their ability to understand and recall the concepts and facts. This ensures a fundamental understanding of medical theory for their future clinical practice. Evaluation of psychomotor domain is performed by practical examinations. Here, the skills of the candidates are assessed by demonstration of clinical examinations, procedures and their ability to use medical instruments. The evaluator is also able to assess the examinee's communication skills, attitude and the ability to apply theoretical knowledge in real-world situations. The viva voce complements theory and practical examinations by providing a near-complete assessment of students' capabilities.

The viva voce examination is a vital component of our assessment system during medical/dental practical examinations in India. The word 'viva voce' is derived from an Ancient Latin word that means 'with a living voice'. Viva voce is an examination process in which the examiner asks questions to the candidate, to which they must reply, usually done in the absence of patients [1]. Their ability to understand and express ideas related to specific topics, reasoning, critical thinking and recall are assessed through the

A. Devadathan (✉)
Pushpagiri Institute of Dental Sciences, Thiruvalla, Kerala, India
Faculty of Dentistry, Kerala University of Health Sciences, Thrissur, Kerala, India
e-mail: dean.dental@kuhs.ac.in

P. R. Rekha
Department of Periodontics, Government Dental College, Kottayam, Kerala, India

R. M. Baiju, S. Thomas (eds.), *The Dental Teacher*,
https://doi.org/10.1007/978-3-032-07551-2_10

direct interaction between the candidate and examiner. Moreover, the viva provides a platform for the examiner to check decision making skills and the professional attitude of students. Viva voce is considered one of the best methods for evaluation of the cognitive domain of the candidate, on any subject because the examiner can evaluate the basic concepts, moving steadily higher and deeper into the topic and finally the current situation or state of research. The examiner can readily rank the student on where he fits on the scale based on his performance. Further, the popularity of viva voce is because the evaluator can assess the knowledge that a candidate has acquired on any topic in a short period of time compared to other methods of assessment.

The viva voce assessment should have a good correlation and match theory examination to a large extent. Viva has a vital characteristic that it assesses what cannot be assessed by a written examination. Since viva voce specifically assess high level of cognitive and affective domain the scoring of viva is more difficult than theory. The question should follow a pattern from a lower level to higher level.

To avoid pitfalls, the evaluator should be aware of the following:

1. Scientific knowledge and clarity in answering is of paramount importance.
2. Logical answering should never be encouraged.
3. Fluency or command over the language shall not be the criterion for awarding marks or credits.

10.2 Characteristics of Good Viva

An ideal viva voce session satisfies the students as well and uplifts their self-esteem and self-confidence. This is possible only when this tool is used thoughtfully, rationally, and objectively. Validity, reliability and fairness are the ideal characteristics of a good viva [2].

10.2.1 Validity

The validity of a viva examination refers to the extent to which it accurately measures the knowledge, skills and competencies it is intended to assess or the ability of the assessment process that allows the candidate to express the extent of their knowledge [3]. To ensure validity the questions being asked in the viva should be within the confines of the content and learning outcomes that need to be tested. This refers to content validity. Construct validity refers to the extent to which the viva examination measures the underlying concepts. A well-conducted viva examination is able to predict the future performance and outcomes and this is called criterion validity. Content validity is ensured with blueprinting, which involves creating a detailed plan and structure of the assessment based on the curriculum.

Blueprinting involves:

1. Clearly defining the purpose and objectives of the viva.
2. Identify the learning outcomes to be tested.

3. Determine the viva format and structure.
4. Prepare clear, concise and unambiguous questions and give proper weightage.
5. Establish a clear assessment criteria aligned with learning outcomes.
6. Define and grade the standards of student performance.

10.2.2 Reliability

The conclusions made from viva assessment should be reliable. If a candidate is tested in a different scenario at a different time by same or another examiner, if he/she gets the same score then the viva can be considered as reliable. They can be termed as intra-rater and inter-rater reliability. In other words, reliability is the extent to which viva produces consistent and dependable results.

10.2.3 Factors Affecting Reliability

1. *Examiner variability*: Different examiners may have different expectations, assessment criteria, scoring standards and topics of interest.
2. *Quality of Questions and consistency*: Poorly worded questions may create ambiguity and confusion in students and produce inconsistent results.
3. Clear assessment *criteria and examiner calibration*: To have clear assessment criteria is absolutely essential to maintain a reliable viva outcome. The examiners should undergo proper training to assess student performance.
4. To some extent, *environmental factors* like noise, distraction, and discomfort also affect the outcomes of viva and produce unreliable results.

10.2.4 Measures to Enhance Reliability

Reliability can be improved by using the same/similar set of questions for all candidates, standard assessment criteria and a structured marking system and proper examiner training [3]. Examiners need to receive formal training in conducting oral examinations. It is important to monitor variations between examiners and address any discrepancies that arise.

10.2.5 Fairness

Fairness refers to the extent to which the assessment process is impartial, unbiased, and equal for all students. A fair viva examination ensures that students are assessed solely on their knowledge and competencies and skills without any discrimination. Fairness ensures that assessment process gives a chance to perform equally well for all candidates. Equal treatment, transparency, freedom from bias, and respect are the cardinal principles of fairness. The tendency of the examiner not to give extreme marks and to rate everyone as average, around the mean is very common during a viva and this may lead to a false central tendency. When lower or higher scores for particular groups of examinees occur, the possibility of bias should be considered [3]. This should be scrutinised by the authorities, and any probable bias should be addressed.

10.2.6 Measures to Ensure Fairness

- *Clear assessment criteria*—having clear, well defined assessment criteria ensures fairness.
- *Examiner training*—with special emphasis on bias, cultural sensitivity to make them aware of fairness.
- *Independent reviewer*—to have moderator or independent reviewer of viva to keep fairness.
- *Student feedback*—seek student feedback to identify what they feel not fair in the viva or what they feel biased.

10.3 The Process of Viva

Viva should be conducted in a pleasant, calm and peaceful atmosphere which makes the candidate tension-free. There should be at least two members for undergraduate examination. Postgraduate examinations should have no more than four examiners, out of which two should be external examiners [4]. It is preferable that members should have a previous experience in viva or a formal training. The examiners should decide among themselves who will chair the viva. The examiner with maximum experience or seniority is typically in charge of the viva. The examiners should make a detailed plan regarding the number of questions, the nature of questions, expected responses and the allotment of marks before the commencement of viva.

Both the examiner and the candidate should come dressed properly for the examinations; otherwise a wrong interpretation of attitude can be made. It also reflects the importance that the candidate gives for the examination. To make the first impression appreciated, appropriate attire plays a big role. A positive vibe for the conduct of viva voce examinations shall be created by the examiners. To begin the conversation, a greeting of the examiner will help. Examiners should behave in a cordial and friendly manner, which surely relax the candidate. Identification of candidate and the proper marking of the candidate's registration number is very important. Examiners should make sure that candidate is tension-free and not anxious. There should not be any discussion related personal affairs. Time management is absolutely essential, and questions should be introduced without much delay [4]. Open questions should be used to give the candidates the opportunity to demonstrate the extent and depth of their knowledge. Closed, complex, lengthy, hypothetical and leading questions are generally not preferred. Use questions covering a range of topics rather than those limited to a single topic. Every minute distraction like phone calls, visitors, talking between examiners should not be entertained. Examiners should properly listen to the answers and should have a positive body language. Students are interrupted only when they deviate from the topic. Maintain eye contact throughout the process. Every candidate should be asked similar questions, not identical questions [4]. Avoid teaching, contradicting, or harassing the student. Give sufficient time to answer and rephrase the questions previously asked to see whether they are able or unable to answer the same. The chairperson should ensure that no discussion or disagreement between examiners is made in the presence of the candidate [5]. The candidate should not receive any information, either directly or indirectly, about the probable outcome of the viva. Judgements like excellent, good, and poor should not be used. To ensure blind marking, the award of marks shall be done by evaluator 2 when evaluator 1 asks the question. This shall be the standard protocol for all viva voce examinations. Sufficient weightage should be considered for short studies conducted, publications, grants or any other academic achievements. Ideally, the viva should not exceed more than 30 minutes. A brief written record of the total process should be maintained, including the date, time, examiner panel and their comments on viva. Some do's and do nots related to viva examination are given in Table 10.1.

10.3.1 Advantages of Traditional Viva

- Enables assessment of knowledge rapidly, in a short time.
- Facilitates assessment of knowledge over vast/many topics.
- Assessment of knowledge from basics to contemporary is enabled.

Table 10.1 *Dos* and *do nots* in viva voce

Dos
Same set of questions for all to begin with.
Questions ordered as must know, desirable to know, good to know.
Ask questions unambiguously.
Put marks then and there.
Create a conducive, non-threatening environment.
Uniform time for all candidates.
Do nots
Ridiculing, threatening.
Teaching during viva.
Indicating about the outcome of the students' performance.
Questions only from favourite topics.
Not paying attention to the candidates' answer.
Comment on the previous candidates' performance.

10.3.2 Disadvantages of Traditional Viva

There are some potential disadvantages to the conventional, traditional, or unstructured viva [6].

- One biggest drawback of traditional viva is that more importance is given to comparison between students rather than individual abilities and achievements. Individual competencies are seldom reflected in marks; only the general performance of the candidate is considered [7].
- Unreliability due to confounding situational factors, anxiety of the examinee, and inconsistency of the examiners.
- Poor objectivity and validity.
- The inevitable element of subjectivity.
- Candidate factors like appearance, language, accent may influence judgement.
- Mostly tests knowledge/recall.
- The candidate order may influence scoring—there is a marked difference between time allotted and scoring among candidates interviewed at the beginning and towards the end of a long viva session.
- High potential for threatening or ridiculing.
- Tendency of examiner to test what is not known rather than what is known.
- Duration is not uniform—too short for certain candidates.
- Viva usually conducted at the end of the practical examinations, both candidates and examiners feel exhausted.

10.4 Objective Structured Viva Examination (OSVE)

Although Oakley and Hencken (2005) introduced structured viva as a distinct assessment technique, it was first discussed and applied in health professions education as early as Thomas et al. in 1993 and Tutton et al. in 1989 [8–10]. Objective structured viva examination is a method of assessment where pre-determined questions and standardised scoring are used for fair, consistent evaluation of students. Undoubtedly this method reduces variability and minimises examiner bias and subjectivity. The series of pre-set questions in OSVE clearly evaluate student's knowledge, skills and attitudes. It is possible to elicit proper cognitive, problem-solving, interpretative, and decision-making skills of the students by structuring the viva. This will guarantee a greater level of validity, reliability, and objectivity. By incorporating input from all those involved in the teaching process, a group of faculty can construct viva questions [7]. Questions should be prepared from each topic with different difficulty levels to meet the learning objectives. It is preferable that each question be split into two halves, the second half exploring the depth of understanding of the first half. The second one is asked only if the candidate answers the first half.

A large number of viva cards from each section are prepared with carefully worded questions. They should be rechecked among colleagues to make sure they are understandable. The prepared viva cards are categorised according to topics or sections. During the viva session, the candidate randomly selects the viva cards from each section (Table 10.2). The examiner reads the question and repeats if necessary. No hints or clues are given.

OSVE is backed by a checklist for evaluation, which is carefully designed in terms of content and competencies in a given amount of time [11]. The examiners mark the appropriate box on a pre-prepared rating scale after hearing candidate's answers to the questions. Splitting the questions and awarding marks by other examiner further enhances reliability and validity. The examiners should not indicate whether the student answers correctly or not. Each question should be given marks separately at the time of answering and total score is calculated at the end. Each examiner is given same time, same number of questions, with equal marks. This is tabulated separately, which is averaged at the end.

The candidates are individually appraised regarding their performance, particularly during internal examinations with a pre-prepared score chart with the awarded marks and examiners comment. Feedback sessions provide an opportunity for the evaluator to inform the student's performance. Understanding the sections where they did not perform well gives the student a chance to improve. Students are also requested to give feedback regarding the entire viva process and modifications are made before the next one. This positive feedback loop definitely improves the quality and outcomes of the viva.

A well-prepared viva card makes the assessment more objective since the candidate himself selects the questions. Exact assessment is also guaranteed since marks are given after each question. A properly outlined scheme makes the viva more structured and less biased, thus imparting a higher degree of validity and reliability.

10.4.1 Advantages of OSVE

- Better validity, reliability and fairness.
- Wide coverage and a uniformity of questions being asked where they are lacking in traditional viva.
- Here, the student has multiple opportunities to express themselves and biases are minimised.
- Viva-cards ensure objectivity, transparency and fairness of examination and results.
- Structured viva has a potential to assess the higher domains of learning.
- Students' satisfaction level is higher in structured viva since they feel more comfortable, relaxed and confident.[11]

Table 10.2 Sample viva card

Usually contains ten questions
60%—Must know
30%—Desirable to know
10%—Good to know

- It enhances the faith of the students in the assessment process.

10.4.2 Disadvantages of OSVE

- Faculty finds difficulty in terms of implementation because structured viva demands detailed planning, pre-validated well structure questions, manpower and resources. This requires a dedicated faculty team and proper planning [2].
- Often, they require minor modifications after each examination, tailoring them with the theory.
- Allotting marks for individual questions is difficult to standardise.
- Structured viva may create apprehension for students since it may involve higher-level and problem-solving type questions.

10.4.3 Key Points in Implementing OSVE

- Prepare a large number of questions or viva cards covering the entire subject, with varying difficulty level. Questions are marked as must-know, desirable-to-know and good-to-know.
- It is better to divide each question into two halves, the second half exploring the depth of the first.
- Validation of questions in each viva card by at least three subject experts for content and relevance.
- Weighting of questions from each section, mark distribution for each question according to their difficulty level, clinical and practical importance.
- Clear guidelines for examiners to assess student response to minimise bias.
- Pilot testing the viva cards in a small group of students.
- Collect feedback from both examiners and examinees.
- Modifications based on the feedback comments.
- Proper training of examiners to familiarise themselves with OSVE.
- Proper student preparation to attend OSVE.

10.4.4 Literature Review of Traditional Viva vs. OSVE

A pilot study conducted by Dhasmana et al. in 2016 on introducing structured viva in medical undergraduate pharmacology suggested that structured viva is a more realistic approach compared to traditional viva and is favoured by most students [7]. A randomised double-blind comparative evaluation done by Imran et al. concluded that structured viva examination provides a uniform, equitable, unbiased and reflective assessment of students [12]. Another comparative study by Dangre-mudey G. et al. in 2016 concluded objective structured viva voce increases objectivity and reduces subjectivity compared to traditional viva [13]. A systematic review and meta-analysis by Anbarasi et al. published in 2022 concluded there is no difference in the mean marks scored by conventional oral and structured oral examination. But structured oral examination will allow examiners to assess the medical students' learning achievement without partiality, stress and anxiety compared to conventional oral examination [11]. Another systematic review and meta-analysis published in 2023 by Abuzied et al. concluded that structured viva has high levels of validity, reliability and acceptability as an assessment tool in health professions education compared to traditional viva [14].

10.5 Conclusions

Viva is a powerful assessment tool if used with proper planning. But inevitably, this process ends with a lot of subjectivity. To overcome this, well-planned objective structured viva examinations should be made mandatory for assessment in medical education. Periodic rechecking and sufficient resources should be deployed by the respective authorities to ensure the candidates coming out through these examinations are competent enough to work in the health sector.

References

1. Cox KR. How to improve oral examinations. Med J Aust. 1978;2(10):176–7.
2. Moleyar VS. How to conduct medical viva. Med J Dr DY Patil Vidyapeeth. 2018;11(4):374–8.
3. Evans LR, Ingersoll RW, Smith EJ. The reliability, validity, and taxonomic structure of the oral examination. J Med Educ. 1966;41:651–7.
4. Shenwai MR, Patil KB. Introduction of structured oral examination as a novel assessment tool to first year medical students in physiology. J Clin Diagn Res. 2013;7:2544–7.
5. Thomas CS, Mellsop G, Callender K, Crawshaw J, Ellis PM, Hall A, et al. The oral examination: a study of academic and non-academic factors. Med Educ. 1993;27:433–9.
6. Davis MH, Karunathilake I. The place of the oral examination in today's assessment systems. Med Teach. 2005;27(4):294–7.
7. Dhasmana DC, Bala S, Sharma R, Sharma T, Kohli S, Aggarwal N, Kalra J. Introducing structured viva voce examination in medical undergraduate pharmacology: a pilot study. Indian J Pharmacol. 2016;48(Suppl 1):S52–6.
8. Oakley B, Hencken C. Oral examination assessment practices: effectiveness and change with a first year undergraduate cohort. J Hosp Leis Sport Tour Educ. 2005;4:3–14.
9. Thomas CS, Mellsop G, Callender K, Crawshaw J, Ellis PM, Hall A, et al. The oral examination: a study of academic and non-academic factors. Med Educ. 1993;27(5):433–9.
10. Tutton PJM, Glasgow EF. Reliability and predictive capacity of examinations in anatomy and improvement in the reliability of viva voce (oral) examinations by the use of a structured rating system. Clin Anat. 1989;21:29–34.
11. Anbarasi K, Karunakaran J, Arthi B, Ravichandran L. Effectiveness of the structured and conventional methods of viva examination in medical education: a systematic review and meta-analysis. J Clin Diagn Res. 2022;16(9)
12. Imran M, Doshi C, Kharadi D. Structured and unstructured viva voce assessment: a double-blind, randomized, comparative evaluation of medical students. Int J Health Sci (Qassim). 2019;13(2):3–9.

13. Dangre-mudey G, Mudey A, Khapre M, Fule S. Performance of undergraduate medical students: traditional viva voce v/s objectively structured viva-voce. J Community Health Manag. 2016;3(2):70–4.
14. Abuzied AIH, Nabag WOM. Structured viva validity, reliability, and acceptability as an assessment tool in health professions education: a systematic review and meta-analysis. BMC Med Educ. 2023;23:531–8.

Objective Structured Clinical Examination (OSCE) in Dentistry

11

Vivek Narayan

11.1 Background

Selecting the appropriate tool from a variety of examination types is both challenging and fascinating. Whilst there is no single 'ideal' examination method for assessing every situation, each tool has its own strengths and limitations in evaluating specific learning domains. For instance, written exams and multiple-choice questions are well-suited for assessing cognitive skills but are less effective for evaluating the psychomotor domain [1].

In the context of dental education, assessing the psychomotor domain of *Bloom's Taxonomy* holds particular importance. Dentistry is inherently a surgical specialty, involving a wide range of procedures—from simple to highly complex—that form the foundation of effective therapy. To succeed, dental surgeons must acquire and demonstrate proficiency in these practical skills. Traditionally, practical examinations have relied on long cases, short cases, and viva voce methods. In long case examinations, candidates are required to take a medical history and conduct a comprehensive physical examination or perform a specific treatment step on a real patient. Specialties such as Oral Medicine, Periodontology, and Orthodontics focus on thorough clinical examinations, diagnosis, and treatment planning. Conversely, fields like Prosthodontics, Conservative Dentistry, and Oral & Maxillofacial Surgery emphasise performing specific procedures, such as making a final impression, completing a Class II restoration, or carrying out a straightforward dental extraction. Candidates are often assigned patients with varying conditions during different examination sessions. They must complete the task within 30–45 min, typically without direct observation by examiners. Following this, unstructured questioning—centred on clinical findings, diagnosis, and patient management—takes place.

V. Narayan (✉)
Public Health Dentistry, Government Dental College, Kottayam, Kerala, India

Kerala University of Health Sciences, Thrissur, Kerala, India

R. M. Baiju, S. Thomas (eds.), *The Dental Teacher*,
https://doi.org/10.1007/978-3-032-07551-2_11

However, critical aspects such as patient interaction, history taking, communication, and clinical skills are frequently unobserved. The focus remains on theoretical knowledge and the proposed management plan rather than practical execution.

The ethical concerns associated with using real patients in undergraduate examinations have often been overlooked. Patients endure significant inconvenience during these assessments. Moreover, variations in patient conditions undermine the reliability and validity of these examinations. A single case limits the ability to evaluate candidates across a spectrum of skills, thereby narrowing the scope of assessment. For example, an excessive emphasis on making an edentulous final impression on the examination day may prevent the evaluation of other essential competencies in Prosthodontics.

Another drawback of long case examinations is the reliance on unstructured questioning rather than standardised checklists or scoring sheets. Despite these challenges, long case exams retain high 'face validity'. The realistic interaction between candidates and patients mirrors actual clinical practice, making these examinations a valuable, albeit imperfect tool. OSCE's were introduced to introduce standardisation and reduce the number of variables that could impact the assessment of performance. Thus, they are considered a better alternative to long case examinations [2, 3].

11.2 Defining an OSCE

An assessment tool based on the principles of objectivity and standardisation, in which candidates move through a series of time-limited stations in a circuit for the purposes of assessing professional performance in a simulated environment. At each station, candidates are assessed and marked against standardised scoring rubrics by trained assessors [2, 3].

Whilst the OSCE focuses on clinical skills like patient interaction, diagnosis, and treatment planning, the OSPE (Objective Structured Practical Examination) emphasises practical skills and lab-based competencies rather than direct patient care [1].

11.3 Evolution of OSCE as an Examination Tool

The first Objective Structured Clinical Examination (OSCE) was introduced by Harden in 1972 in Dundee [2]. In its original format, students rotated through 18 testing stations and two rest stations within a hospital ward. Each station lasted 4.5 min, with a 30-s break between them, making the total examination time 100 min. Each station focused on assessing a specific competency, such as performing a procedure, taking a patient's history, or conducting a clinical examination.

Over time, the OSCE has gained widespread acceptance as the preferred method for evaluating clinical competence across various educational stages, medical specialties and regions worldwide. It is now regarded as the gold standard for performance assessment, significantly influencing medical education. Today, the OSCE

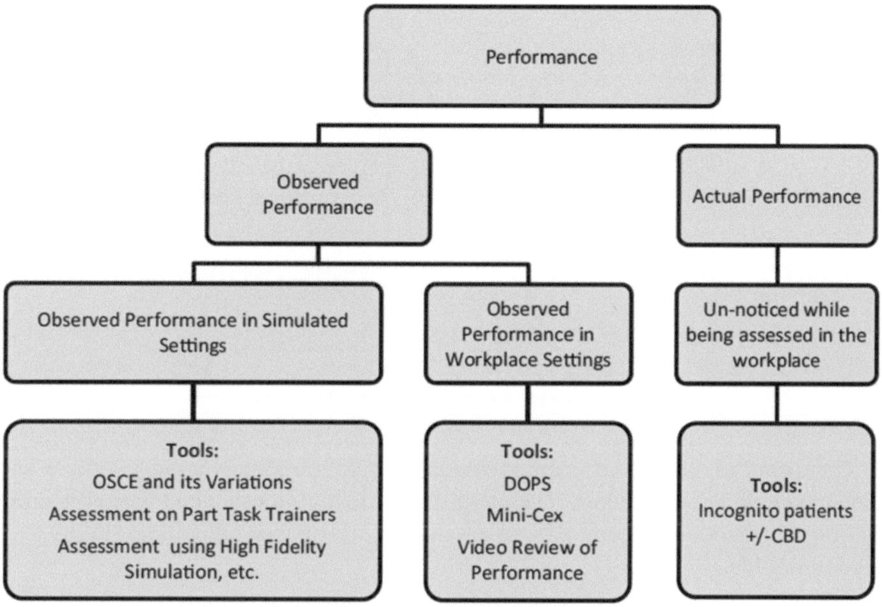

Fig. 11.1 Assessment methods for professional performance [4]

primarily serves as a tool for evaluating clinical skills in simulated settings. However, other methods are available for assessing performance in real-world clinical environments as shown in Fig. 11.1 [3].

It is important to remember that the simulated environment can impact candidates' performance, meaning their results in the OSCE may not fully reflect how they would perform the same tasks in a real workplace setting. In real-life settings, non-clinical skills such as teamwork, resource management, situational awareness, and leadership play a crucial role in overall performance. However, these skills are challenging to assess effectively through the OSCE. The OSCEs are therefore better aligned with the 'Shows how' compartment of the *Miller's Pyramid* rather than the 'Does' compartment.

11.4 Principles of OSCE Assessment

OSCE tests demonstration of competence under supervision (Fig. 11.2). The OSCE is built on two key principles: objectivity and structure. Objectivity relies on standardised scoring rubrics and ensures that a trained examiner asks the same questions to all candidates. Structure, on the other hand, involves a standardised station design that assesses a specific clinical task, aligned with the curriculum blueprint. A well-designed OSCE demonstrates a high level of validity. It has been demonstrated that reliability and validity improve by increasing the number of stations, having trained examiners and also by using standardised rubrics [2, 5, 6].

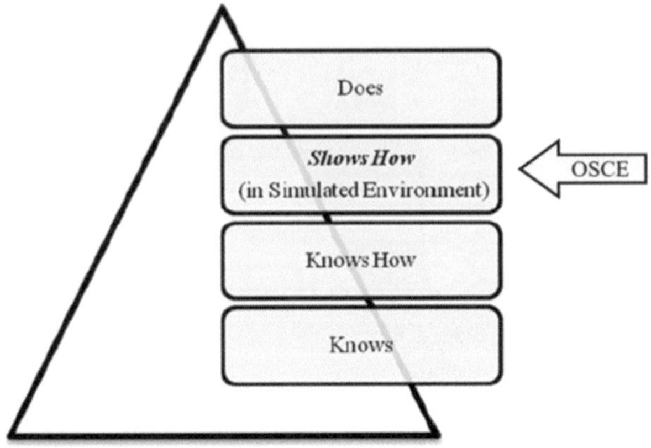

Fig. 11.2 *Miller's Pyramid* for assessment [1, 3]

Compared to other assessment methods, the OSCE requires more resources and time to set up and administer. Therefore, it is essential to use the OSCE efficiently by designing stations specifically for assessing performance rather than simply testing knowledge.

The OSCE can positively influence education by promoting learning. This impact depends on how accurately assessment scenarios are recreated at OSCE stations. When candidates perceive little difference between OSCE tasks and real-life practice, the exam encourages lifelong learning. However, if tasks are overly compartmentalised and rely heavily on checklist-based scoring, candidates may focus solely on passing the exam, thereby reducing the OSCE's overall educational value [5, 7].

11.5 Setting up an OSCE

1. **Blueprint Development.**

   Blueprinting is the structured process of defining the content of an examination. In the context of an OSCE, it involves selecting the range of skills to be assessed and determining how frequently each skill appears in the exam. The OSCE/OSPE stations have to be selected carefully ensuring that the assessment aligns well with the objectives laid out in the curriculum.
2. **OSCE Stations.**

   An OSCE circuit typically consists of the following types of stations [2, 3]:

   (a) **Observed Stations:** An examiner is present throughout the station to assess the candidate's performance in clinical examination, procedures, or communication skills. The examiners will rate the performance of each candidate using a standardised scoring checklist/rubric/rating scale.

   (b) **Unobserved Stations**: No examiner is present during these stations. Candidates submit their responses on paper either after each station or at the end of the exam. These stations assess skills such as interpreting clinical information (e.g., X-rays, pathology specimens, blood results), prescribing, or IT-related tasks. The student may also be asked to answer objective type questions.

(c) **Linked Stations**: Two consecutive stations based on the same clinical scenario. These may be observed or unobserved. For example, a candidate might perform a clinical examination of the temporomandibular joint in one-station and document findings with a management plan in the next.

OSCE stations may use real patients, standardised patients (actors), or simulation equipment, including models, task trainers, and high-fidelity mannequins, to create a realistic clinical environment.

3. **OSCE Circuit and Station Setup**

Students rotate through stations, completing practical tasks or solving problems designed to assess specific skills. Stations may be set up in multiple small rooms, resembling outpatient clinics, or in a larger space divided into designated station areas using screens. The OSCE circuit refers to the structured arrangement of stations that ensures a seamless flow of candidates. Each candidate progresses individually through all stations during the exam. To maintain efficiency, the number of candidates per sitting should match the number of stations unless rest stations are included.

4. **OSCE Assessment and Standard Setting**

Examiners evaluate students using **predefined criteria**, typically through checklists or rating scales. The assessment is objective, focusing on observable and measurable skills.

Checklists and Rating Scales

- **Checklists**: List specific actions expected at a station. They can be:
  - **Binary (Yes/No):** Indicating whether an action was performed or not.
  - **Rating Scales (5–7 Points):** Allowing assessment based on the quality of performance.
- **Global Rating Scales**: Unlike task-specific checklists, these assess the overall process, making them more suitable for evaluating skills where quality is as important as completion. They are particularly useful for assessing judgment, empathy, organisation of knowledge, and technical skills.

Standard Setting

Standard setting defines the passing score for candidates. There are two main methods [6]:

1. **Norm-Referenced Methods**: Scores are interpreted relative to other candidates, with pass/fail thresholds based on comparative performance.
2. **Criterion-Referenced Methods**: A predefined standard is set, below which a candidate is deemed unfit to practice. Scores have absolute meanings tied to specific competencies. Common approaches include:
   - Angoff Method (1971).
   - Ebel Method (1972).

5. **Feedback in OSCE**

Immediate feedback may be given to candidates at each station or collectively in a post-examination session. Examiner feedback on the examination process helps improve station quality and the overall organisation of future OSCEs. Additionally, candidates may be invited to share their experiences as part of the quality assurance process [2, 6].

11.6 Advantages of OSCE

The OSCE offers several advantages as an assessment tool [2, 6, 8]. It provides an objective and standardised evaluation by minimising examiner bias through structured checklists and predefined criteria. This ensures that every candidate is assessed under the same conditions. OSCE is potentially highly comprehensive, testing a wide range of skills, including clinical examination, procedural tasks, communication, decision-making, professionalism, and teamwork. By simulating real-world patient interactions, it helps students develop clinical readiness and encourages active learning. Another key benefit is the provision of immediate and constructive feedback, allowing candidates to reflect on their performance and improve their skills. OSCE is also flexible and adaptable, as stations can be tailored to assess different levels of competency across various medical specialties. Furthermore, its structured approach enhances fairness and reproducibility, reducing variability in assessment outcomes. Lastly, the format motivates students to engage in systematic skill development, reinforcing both theoretical and practical knowledge.

11.7 Limitations of OSCE

Despite its advantages, OSCE has limitations in terms of objectivity, validity, and reliability, particularly in resource-poor settings. It is both costly and time-consuming, requiring significant effort and investment to design stations that effectively assess key professional competencies, such as teamwork, ethical behavior, and self-appraisal [5, 7].

11.8 Conclusion

The often-used phrase 'assessment drives learning' is particularly relevant to OSCE. A well-structured OSCE ensures that students focus on acquiring clinical competencies, problem-solving abilities, and practical skills rather than just memorising theoretical knowledge. OSCEs have stood the test of time as a valid and unbiased tool for objective assessment in medical education. However, significant challenges hinder their routine implementation, particularly in resource-poor settings. In such environments, medical educators often juggle multiple roles—as clinicians, researchers, and administrators—leaving little time for the meticulous planning and execution that an effective OSCE requires. As a result, OSCEs in these settings risk becoming mere formalities rather than true assessments of clinical competence.

References

1. Medical Council of India. Assessment module for undergraduate medical education training program; 2019
2. Harden RM, Lilley P, Patrício M. The definitive guide to the OSCE. Elsiever; 2016.
3. Khan KZ, Ramachandran S, Gaunt K, Pushkar P. The objective structured clinical examination (OSCE): AMEE guide no. 81. Part I: an historical and theoretical perspective. Med Teach. 2013;35(9):e1437–46. https://doi.org/10.3109/0142159X.2013.818634.
4. Khan K, Ramachandran S. Conceptual framework for performance assessment: competency, competence and performance in the context of assessments in healthcare—deciphering the terminology. Med Teach. 2012;34(11):920–8.
5. Barman A. Critiques on the objective structured clinical examination. Ann Acad Med Singap. 2005;34(8):478–82.
6. Khan KZ, Gaunt K, Ramachandran S, Pushkar P. The objective structured clinical examination (OSCE): AMEE guide no. 81. Part II: organisation & administration. Med Teach. 2013;35(9):e1447–63. https://doi.org/10.3109/0142159X.2013.818635.
7. Gupta P, Dewan P, Singh T. Objective structured clinical examination (OSCE) revisited. Indian Pediatr. 2010;47(11):911–20. https://doi.org/10.1007/s13312-010-0155-6.
8. Puryer J. Dental undergraduate views of objective structured clinical examinations (OSCEs): a literature review. Dent J. 2016;4(1):6. https://doi.org/10.3390/dj4010006.

12 Long-Case and Short-Case Assessment in Dental Education

N. D. Jayakumar and Nidhitha Suresh

12.1 Introduction

12.1.1 History Taking and Clinical Case Discussion in Dental Practice

History taking and clinical examination are fundamental components of medical and dental practice, forming the cornerstone of accurate diagnosis and effective patient management. These skills are rigorously taught and assessed at both undergraduate and postgraduate levels, emphasising their pivotal role in healthcare delivery [1].

12.1.2 The Significance of History Taking

Thomas Sydenham's statement that '*Watching a patient and interacting with him can reveal more than any examination could*' highlights the crucial role of history taking in clinical practice. This process involves systematically collecting comprehensive information about a patient's medical history, symptoms, and lifestyle, offering valuable insights into their overall health and potential risk factors.

Despite significant advancements in diagnostic technologies and therapeutic approaches, history taking remains an essential pillar of patient care. It not only facilitates accurate diagnosis but also fosters a deeper understanding of the patient as a whole. Moreover, it plays a vital role in establishing trust—a fundamental aspect of the patient-physician relationship. A trusting rapport enhances the effectiveness of clinical encounters, encourages open communication, and helps alleviate patient anxiety, ultimately improving the overall healthcare experience.

N. D. Jayakumar (✉) · N. Suresh
Saveetha University, Chennai, India

R. M. Baiju, S. Thomas (eds.), *The Dental Teacher*,
https://doi.org/10.1007/978-3-032-07551-2_12

As medical practice evolves with improved diagnostics and widespread access to medical information, the patient-physician dynamic has shifted towards shared decision-making. This collaborative approach underscores the enduring importance of history taking, as it strengthens communication and trust, ensuring more patient-centred and effective care [2].

12.1.3 The Importance of Clinical Examination

Clinical examination plays a crucial role in patient assessment, with its primary objectives being to *identify the etiological agents responsible for the disease, determine its severity, and establish an accurate diagnosis* to develop an effective treatment plan. Whilst history taking provides valuable insights into a patient's condition, clinical examination complements it by allowing healthcare professionals to detect physical signs that may not be apparent through history alone. Mastery of this skill enables practitioners to recognise subtle clinical indicators, guide further diagnostic investigations, and implement timely interventions, ultimately improving patient outcomes [3].

12.2 Relevance in Dental Practice

In dental practice, history taking and clinical examination are equally critical. A comprehensive patient history and meticulous clinical examination are essential for diagnosing oral diseases, formulating treatment plans, and predicting outcomes. For example, understanding a patient's medication history is crucial in periodontal care since medications such as antihypertensives, anticonvulsants, and immunosuppressants can influence periodontal health through diverse mechanisms. These include genetic predisposition, fibroblast proliferation, inhibited cation flux, reduced folate uptake, impaired collagenase activation, inflammatory cytokine elevation, and plaque-induced inflammation [4].

By combining detailed history taking with skilled clinical examination, healthcare professionals can ensure a precise diagnosis and effective patient-centred care, highlighting the timeless relevance of these foundational practices in the field of dentistry.

12.3 Patient Interaction and Communication in Periodontal Care

Effective patient interaction and communication are fundamental in the management of periodontitis, as they lay the groundwork for accurate diagnosis, treatment planning, and adherence to therapeutic regimens. Building rapport and establishing trust are critical in encouraging patients to share sensitive information about their oral and systemic health. This relationship fosters open communication and helps *alleviate patient anxiety*, making the clinical process more efficient and patient-centred [5].

Cultural sensitivity and empathy are particularly important when addressing periodontitis, as patients may come from diverse backgrounds with varying beliefs about oral health. Understanding and respecting these perspectives enable clinicians to deliver personalised care, thereby enhancing patient satisfaction and compliance with treatment recommendations.

12.4 Components of a Comprehensive History in Periodontal Care

A thorough history is indispensable in diagnosing and managing periodontitis. The key components include:

1. **Chief Complaint**
   A patient presenting with periodontal issues, such as bleeding gums, loose teeth, bad breath, or swollen gums, offers a focused starting point for evaluation.
2. **History of Present Illness**
   It is crucial to gather detailed information about the onset, duration, progression, and associated symptoms of periodontal issues. This includes identifying potential triggers such as alterations in oral hygiene practices, systemic conditions, or factors like stress that may contribute to the condition.
3. **Past Medical and Dental History**
   Exploring the patient's medical history is crucial to identify systemic conditions (e.g. diabetes, cardiovascular diseases) that exacerbate periodontitis. Similarly, dental history, including previous periodontal treatments, oral hygiene practices, and habits like bruxism, provides insight into disease progression and risk factors.
4. **Family History, Social History, and Lifestyle Factors**

Understanding a patient's family history, social background, and lifestyle factors is essential for assessing risks contributing to periodontal disease. Genetic predispositions, along with habits such as smoking, alcohol use, and dietary choices, have a significant impact on periodontal health. In this context, macronutrients play a crucial role—high sugar intake can cause microbiota dysbiosis, thereby increasing periodontal disease risk, whilst fibre and polyols offer protective effects. Fats, particularly saturated fatty acids, contribute to oxidative stress, whilst omega-3 fatty acids have anti-inflammatory benefits. Micronutrients like vitamins A, C, D, and calcium are crucial, with deficiencies linked to periodontal diseases. Polyphenols and probiotics also support periodontal health, though prebiotic evidence is still limited [6]. Furthermore, social factors such as access to dental care and stress levels are vital in crafting an effective treatment plan. Ultimately, a balanced diet plays a significant role in preventing and managing periodontal diseases.

12.5 Key Components Involved in Clinical Examination

A thorough clinical examination is fundamental for diagnosing and managing periodontitis, providing essential insights into a patient's oral health and guiding treatment planning. This process requires a systematic and consistent approach, along with strict adherence to infection control protocols to ensure the safety of both the patient and the clinician. Creating a comfortable environment is equally important to encourage patient cooperation and reduce anxiety during the examination.

The assessment begins with an extraoral examination, which includes evaluating facial symmetry, inspecting skin lesions, and palpating lymph nodes to detect potential systemic or localised abnormalities. This is followed by a comprehensive intraoral examination, focusing on the oral mucosa, teeth, periodontal tissues, and occlusion. It is essential to carefully evaluate gingival health by examining signs of inflammation, such as redness and swelling, along with assessing gingival colour, contour, consistency, and surface texture. *Whilst bleeding on probing (BOP) is a widely used indicator, its accuracy can be inconsistent due to variations in technique, probe type, and site-specific factors.* Probing the marginal gingiva is generally more reliable but may sometimes yield false-positive results due to trauma. Careful observation of gingival contour and architecture is essential, particularly noting the 'knifelike' appearance of the free marginal gingiva and its pyramidal form supported by the subgingival cervical ridge of enamel.

Measuring probing depths is crucial for detecting periodontal pockets and assessing attachment loss, whilst gingival recession serves as a marker for advanced periodontal damage. Diagnostic tools, including dental mirrors, periodontal probes, and radiographs, are indispensable for obtaining comprehensive clinical data such as pocket depths, clinical attachment levels, and bone loss. Radiographic assessments, including intraoral periapical radiographs, bitewing radiographs, orthopantomograms (OPGs), and Cone-Beam Computed Tomography (CBCT), are crucial for visualising bone and soft tissue structures. These imaging techniques facilitate accurate diagnosis and help guide informed treatment planning.

Comprehensive periodontal charting, which includes probing depths, furcation involvement, tooth mobility, and radiographic interpretations, is vital for establishing baselines and monitoring disease progression. Tooth mobility is a crucial parameter in periodontal assessment and can occur with or without gingival inflammation. Whilst periodontal disease is a major cause, several other factors can also contribute to tooth mobility. These include occlusal trauma, which leads to the widening of the periodontal ligament, as well as endodontic or traumatic influences. Anatomical considerations, such as unfavourable root morphology (e.g. short or tapering roots), can further exacerbate mobility. By integrating these factors, clinicians can achieve a comprehensive and dynamic assessment, leading to accurate diagnoses and personalised, effective periodontal care [7].

12.6 An Innovative Approach to a Comprehensive History and Clinical Examination for Patients with Bleeding Gums: A Guide to Effective Diagnosis and Treatment Planning

12.6.1 Chief Complaint

1. How long have you noticed bleeding gums?

The question **'How long have you noticed bleeding gums?'** is useful for assessing the duration and severity of the condition, offering valuable insight into potential underlying causes. Chronic or persistent gum bleeding may indicate systemic disorders such as leukaemia, where thrombocytopenia and increased vascular fragility contribute to excessive bleeding. Bleeding disorders like haemophilia and von Willebrand disease, as well as vitamin deficiencies (e.g., Vitamin C deficiency leading to scurvy or Vitamin K deficiency affecting clotting), can also cause prolonged gum bleeding. Vitamin C deficiency disrupts collagen synthesis and increases capillary fragility, whilst Vitamin K deficiency impairs clotting factor production, reducing the blood's ability to form clots and making gums more prone to bleeding. Additionally, liver disease (such as cirrhosis) can affect clotting factor production, further contributing to excessive bleeding.

Sudden gingival bleeding may indicate a medication-related cause, especially due to anticoagulants or antiplatelet drugs. It may also indicate autoimmune diseases like Wegener's granulomatosis or vasculitis, which affect blood vessel integrity and increase bleeding susceptibility. Additionally, sudden unexplained bleeding should raise suspicion of drug-induced thrombocytopenia (DIT), particularly in patients taking medications. DIT can further compromise platelet function, exacerbating bleeding tendencies. It is important to consider the patient's medication history to identify any potential drugs contributing to thrombocytopenia and bleeding.

2. Is the bleeding spontaneous, or does it occur during brushing or flossing?

Understanding whether the bleeding is spontaneous or triggered by activities like brushing, flossing, or eating can help differentiate the underlying cause. One distinguishing feature of spontaneous gingival bleeding is the occurrence of bleeding without provocation, which may even manifest during sleep. Patients often report waking up to find their pillows stained or wet with blood. Recognising this sign during patient history-taking and clinical examination is essential for accurate diagnosis and appropriate management. Spontaneous bleeding may indicate more serious systemic conditions, such as leukaemia, bleeding disorders, or autoimmune diseases, where there is a more generalised issue with blood clotting or vessel fragility. On the other hand, if the bleeding occurs primarily during brushing or flossing, it is more likely associated with gingivitis, periodontitis, or localised trauma to the gums. This distinction helps in narrowing down whether the issue is isolated to oral health or potentially linked to a broader systemic condition.

3. Do you have any other concerns, such as bad breath, loose teeth, or swollen gums?

Additional symptoms, such as bad breath (halitosis), loose teeth, and swollen gums, can provide important clues to underlying conditions. *Bad breath* may be a sign of periodontal disease, poor oral hygiene, or oral candidiasis. It can also indicate systemic conditions like diabetes (fruity breath in ketoacidosis) or liver disease. *Loose teeth* often point to advanced periodontitis or osteoporosis, and can be linked to systemic diseases that affect bone metabolism, such as diabetes or hyperparathyroidism. Malignancies like leukaemia that affect bone marrow health can also lead to loose teeth. *Swollen gums* can result from gingivitis, periodontitis, or vitamin C deficiency (scurvy), as well as drug-induced gingival overgrowth (such as from phenytoin, cyclosporine, or calcium channel blockers). In some cases, swollen gums may be associated with leukaemia or other systemic inflammatory conditions. These symptoms help narrow down the potential causes, whether they are localised oral issues or indicative of more serious systemic diseases.

12.6.2 History of Present Illness

1. Have you noticed bleeding in other areas, such as the nose (epistaxis), skin bruising, or blood in urine/stool?

The question, 'Have you noticed bleeding in other areas, such as the nose (epistaxis), skin bruising, or blood in urine/stool?' It is important for identifying potential systemic causes of bleeding gums. If the patient reports bleeding in areas beyond the gums, it suggests the possibility of a broader underlying issue, such as a hematologic or systemic disorder. For example, epistaxis (nosebleeds) can be associated with platelet dysfunction or vascular fragility, commonly seen in conditions like leukaemia, thrombocytopenia, or von Willebrand disease. Unexplained skin bruising may indicate bleeding disorders like haemophilia, vitamin K deficiency, or liver disease, all of which affect clotting factors. Additionally, blood in the urine (haematuria) or stool (melena/hematochezia) could suggest systemic bleeding disorders or gastrointestinal bleeding, which are often exacerbated by clotting abnormalities seen in conditions like haemophilia, liver disease, or disseminated intravascular coagulation (DIC). When bleeding is reported in multiple areas, it raises suspicion for a systemic bleeding disorder, prompting further haematological investigations (e.g. CBC, coagulation profile, liver function tests) to differentiate between localised gingival problems and more serious systemic conditions such as leukaemia, vitamin deficiencies, or bleeding disorders that may require specialised treatment.

2. Have you recently changed your oral hygiene practices, such as using a new toothbrush or toothpaste?

The question 'Have you recently changed your oral hygiene practises, such as using a new toothbrush or toothpaste? It is important to diagnose the cause of bleeding gums, as changes in oral care habits can significantly impact gum health. If a patient reports bleeding gums and has recently switched to a new toothbrush or toothpaste, it may indicate that the change is either causing or contributing to the issue. For example, using a new toothbrush with hard bristles or improper brushing technique can lead to mechanical irritation of the gums, resulting in bleeding, especially if the gums are already inflamed from gingivitis or periodontal disease. If the toothpaste contains allergens or harsh chemicals, it may trigger a reaction that leads to bleeding. A recent change in brushing routine, such as an increase in brushing frequency or intensity, may also irritate the gums, especially if the patient has an existing gum infection. Understanding these factors helps pinpoint whether the bleeding is due to improper oral hygiene habits or an underlying condition.

12.7 Past Medical and Dental History

Questions regarding a patient's past medical and dental history are essential in diagnosing the cause of bleeding gums and determining whether it is related to oral health or systemic conditions. Asking about systemic health issues such as diabetes, cardiovascular disease, liver disease, or autoimmune disorders helps identify underlying conditions that may contribute to gum bleeding. Inquiring about medications, especially blood thinners like aspirin or warfarin, is crucial as they can increase the risk of bleeding, including in the gums. Additionally, asking about any recent use of medications that could potentially cause drug-induced thrombocytopenia (DIT) is important, as DIT can exacerbate bleeding tendencies. A thorough medical history, including all medications (prescription, over-the-counter, non-conventional therapies, and herbal remedies), is necessary, with special attention to high-risk drugs like quinine and sulfonamides. DIT is often confirmed when platelet counts recover after discontinuing a suspected drug. Other causes of thrombocytopenia, such as sepsis, disseminated intravascular coagulation (DIC), thrombotic thrombocytopenic purpura (TTP), and heparin-induced thrombocytopenia (HIT), should also be considered. Immune thrombocytopenic purpura (ITP) and thrombocytopenia in HIV patients are additional possibilities. Proper evaluation ensures accurate diagnosis and effective treatment [8].

Aspirin, a non-steroidal anti-inflammatory drug (NSAID), contributes to gingival bleeding due to its antiplatelet effects, impairing platelet aggregation and prolonging bleeding time. The gingiva, rich in capillaries, is particularly vulnerable to bleeding, especially when inflammation progresses to gingivitis [9]. Additionally, Vitamin K deficiency, which impairs clotting factor production, can also contribute to gingival bleeding by further reducing the ability to form clots. In individuals with gingivitis or periodontitis, these factors elevate the risk of prolonged bleeding. The patient's history of periodontal treatments and frequency of dental visits also provide insight into whether the bleeding is related to recurring periodontal issues or a new condition. These questions help the clinician determine whether the bleeding is localised to the gums or indicative of broader systemic health concerns.

12.8 Family History

The questions regarding family history are important for identifying potential genetic or hereditary factors that could contribute to bleeding gums. Asking if there is a family history of periodontal disease, bleeding disorders, diabetes, or other systemic conditions helps to uncover any genetic predisposition to these issues, which can increase the likelihood of similar problems occurring in the patient. Inquiring whether close family members have experienced similar symptoms, such as bleeding gums or tooth loss, can further indicate a familial pattern of oral health issues or systemic conditions that might be contributing to the patient's symptoms. This information is crucial for identifying potential underlying causes and guiding the diagnosis and treatment.

12.9 Clinical Examination

12.9.1 Extra: Oral Examination

The extra-oral examination is essential for identifying signs that may indicate underlying systemic conditions contributing to bleeding gums. Skin lesions or discolouration, such as petechiae, ecchymosis, or jaundice, should be noted as they can point to conditions like bleeding disorders, liver disease, or vasculitis. Palpation of lymph nodes in the head and neck region (including submandibular, cervical, and supraclavicular nodes) helps detect enlargement, tenderness, or abnormal mobility, which could signal infections, malignancies, or systemic conditions affecting gum health. Examination of the lips and commissures is also important for identifying signs of nutritional deficiencies, such as cracking or sores, which could indicate conditions like angular cheilitis due to iron or vitamin deficiencies. Additionally, observing the colour of the skin and sclera for a yellowish discolouration is crucial as it could suggest jaundice, which is often associated with liver dysfunction. Finally, assessing for pallor can indicate anaemia, a condition that may contribute to gum bleeding due to reduced blood oxygenation.

12.9.2 Intraoral Examination

12.9.2.1 Gingival Findings

Gingival Findings: The colour of the gingiva can provide important clues about the patient's health. A bright red or bluish hue often suggests inflammation, commonly seen in conditions like gingivitis or periodontitis, whilst pallor may be a sign of anaemia. A yellowish hue could indicate liver disease. The normal contour of the gingiva is scalloped with knife-edged gingival margins, but flattened or swollen contours may suggest gingival inflammation, periodontitis, or gingival enlargement. This enlargement or change in contour could be due to underlying issues like vitamin deficiencies, systemic diseases, or even due to the use of medications such as those seen with Phenytoin or calcium channel blockers. In patients with systemic conditions such as bleeding disorders, liver disease, or vasculitis, the gingiva often appears oedematous, swollen, and friable, making it highly susceptible to spontaneous bleeding. The colour may vary, with a bright red or bluish hue indicating increased vascular fragility, whilst pallor may suggest anaemia, commonly associated with chronic liver disease. In cases of liver dysfunction, a yellowish hue may be observed due to bilirubin accumulation. The normal knife-edged gingival margins may be replaced by swollen, flattened, or irregular contours, reflecting underlying inflammation or systemic influence. In chronic conditions, the gingiva may become fibrotic rather than oedematous.

Tooth mobility is generally absent unless there is secondary involvement of alveolar bone loss due to osteoporosis or metabolic disorders, where mobility may range from Grade I to III. Furcation involvement is uncommon unless periodontal disease is present, but advanced systemic conditions can contribute to periodontal structural deterioration. The buccal mucosa may exhibit petechiae, ecchymosis, or purpura, particularly in patients with platelet disorders, vasculitis, or coagulation defects. In individuals with liver disease, pallor due to anaemia and jaundice from impaired bilirubin metabolism may also be noticeable. The soft palate is a common site for petechiae and ecchymosis, which are hallmark signs of thrombocytopenia or vasculitis. Likewise, the hard palate may show petechiae, ecchymosis, or purpura, whilst spider angiomas, commonly associated with chronic liver disease due to altered estrogen metabolism, can also occur as a result of pregnancy or oral contraceptive use.

12.10 Differential Diagnosis for a Patient Presenting with a Chief Complaint of Gingival Bleeding

The assessment of clinical acumen derives its foundation at the cognitive domain. In assessment of a student's clinical performance, higher levels of the cognitive domain incorporating applied knowledge are focused upon. In that aspect assigning differential diagnoses assumes importance. The following table plots the approach towards assessing a patient with gingival bleeding (Tables 12.1 and 12.2).

Table 12.1 Possible differential diagnoses for bleeding from gums

Chief complaint	Investigations	Diagnosis
Spontaneous gingival bleeding	Hemoglobin, increased bleeding time, prolonged activated partial thromboplastin time (APTT), abnormal platelet aggregation (with ADP, collagen, epinephrine); prolonged pro- thrombin time	Glanzmann Thrombasthenia
	Decreased platelet count, prolonged bleeding time, normal PT and APTT	Thrombocytopenic Purpura
	Prolonged APTT, normal PT, reduced factor VIII or IX levels	Haemophilia A or B
	Prolonged PT and APTT, decreased fibrinogen levels, increased D-dimer	Disseminated Intravascular Coagulation (DIC)
	Increased bleeding time decreased von Willebrand factor levels, prolonged APTT	von Willebrand disease
	Clinical examination (pallor, petechiae, gingival enlargement), peripheral blood smear, bone marrow biopsy, complete blood count (CBC)	Leukaemia
	Prolonged PT and INR, history of warfarin use	Warfarin-induced coagulopathy
	Low vitamin C levels	Scurvy
	Clinical examination, radiographs (to detect bone loss), probing depth measurement	Chronic periodontitis
	History of systemic diseases, hyperglycemia, clinical examination with probing depth and radiographs showing bone loss	Periodontitis associated with systemic disease
	Ulcerative lesions in the oral mucosa, nosules, infiltrations or cavities on chest radiograph, abnormal urinary sediment, granulomatous inflammation on biopsy, anti-neutrophil cytoplasmic antibody test (ANCA test)	Wegener's granulomatosis
	Sudden onset pain, halitosis, ulceration and necrosis of interdental papilla	Acute necrotizing ulcerative gingivitis

Table 12.2 Decision tree for differential diagnosis of patient reporting with a chief complaint of bleeding gums

Chief Complaint - Bleeding gums

Chronic, Persistent / Spontaneous Bleeding	Sudden onset of Bleeding	Bleeding while brushing / flossing	• Other Associated symptoms
• Leukemia	• Acute Gingival infections-ANUG	• Gingivitis ,Periodontitis	• Bad breath- Periodontal Disease, systemic conditions such as Diabetes , liver disease
• Bleeding Disorders	• Medication induced -Antiplatelet, anticoagulant	• Localized trauma to gingiva	• Loose Teeth- Periodontitis , Leukemia
• Vitamin Deficiencies			• Swollen gums - Medication induced, Periodontitis , Vitamin Deficiency
• Liver Diseases			• Ulceration and necrosis of IDP- ANUG
			• Nose bleeds - Bleeding Disorders, Wegener granulomatosis, leukemia, liver disease

References

1. Singh H, Graber ML. Improving diagnosis in health care—the next imperative for patient safety. New England J Med. 2015;373(26):2493–5.
2. Drake WM, Hutchison R. Hutchison's clinical methods, An integrated approach to clinical practice with STUDENT CONSULT Online Access, 23: Hutchison's Clinical Methods. Elsevier Health Sciences; 2012.
3. Greenwood M. Essentials of medical history-taking in dental patients. Dent Update. 2015;42(4):308-10–313-5. https://doi.org/10.12968/denu.2015.42.4.308.
4. Seymour RA, Heasman PA. Drugs and the periodontium. J Clin Periodontol. 1988;15(1):1–16. https://doi.org/10.1111/j.1600-051x.1988.tb01549.x.
5. Dang BN, Westbrook RA, Njue SM, Giordano TP. Building trust and rapport early in the new doctor-patient relationship: a longitudinal qualitative study. BMC Med Educ. 2017;17(1):32. https://doi.org/10.1186/s12909-017-0868-5. PMID: 28148254; PMCID: PMC5288896.
6. Martinon P, Fraticelli L, Giboreau A, Dussart C, Bourgeois D, Carrouel F. Nutrition as a key modifiable factor for periodontitis and main chronic diseases. J Clin Med. 2021;10(2):197. https://doi.org/10.3390/jcm10020197. PMID: 33430519; PMCID: PMC7827391.
7. Newman MG, Takei H, Klokkevold PR, Carranza FA. Newman and Carranza's clinical periodontology. Elsevier Health Sciences; 2018.
8. George JN, Aster RH. Drug-induced thrombocytopenia: pathogenesis, evaluation, and management. Hematol Am Soc Hematol Educ Program. 2009:153–8. https://doi.org/10.1182/asheducation-2009.1.153. PMID: 20008194; PMCID: PMC4413903.
9. Royzman D,Recio L,Badovinac RL,Fiorellini J,Goodson M,Howell H,Karimbux N. The effect of aspirin intake on bleeding on probing in patients with gingivitis. J Periodontol.2004;75(5):679-684. https://doi.org/10.1902/jop.2004.75.5.679.

13 The Art of Mentoring Dental Students

Vinod Krishnan

13.1 Introduction

Mentoring helps and advises a younger or less experienced person (mentee), particularly in a job or at school (Cambridge Dictionary) [1]. Like various professions, dentistry is witnessing a surge in developing a mentoring culture that promotes and supports personal growth. Increasing awareness shows that becoming an effective dental professional requires outstanding technical skills and strong diagnostic, individual, and motivational competencies. Achieving these objectives necessitates collaboration within a nurturing and supportive professional environment. Mentoring programmes bridge the gap between different levels of expertise and experience, help with mentees' professional development, and reinforce mentors' leadership skills.

13.2 Historical Perspective

The term 'mentor' originates from the character Mentor in Homer's Odyssey. When Odysseus, king of Ithaca, left to fight in the Trojan War, he entrusted his friend Mentor with the responsibility of advising and teaching his son, Telemachus. Over time, the word mentor evolved to describe someone who serves as a guide and educator, with a mentoring relationship viewed as a connection between teacher and student. Whilst mentorship is often idealised as a positive phenomenon, the original Greek interpretations depicted a more nuanced relationship between Mentor and Telemachus [2].

V. Krishnan (✉)
Department of Orthodontics, Sri Sankara Dental College, Thiruvananthapuram, Kerala, India

Kerala University of Health Sciences, Thrissur, Kerala, India

R. M. Baiju, S. Thomas (eds.), *The Dental Teacher*,
https://doi.org/10.1007/978-3-032-07551-2_13

13.3 Mentor and Mentee

13.3.1 Mentor

A mentor is someone with valuable experience and knowledge who offers guidance and support. In mentoring programmes, mentors are guides who help promote professional growth and skill development, and their role is not just limited to that of advisors. They share insights and can open doors that might remain closed to a mentee. They may perform various mentoring functions, sometimes as coaches, connectors, or even challengers, to help their mentees reach their full potential.

Not all mentors are created equal; there are five distinct types [3, 4]:

1. Traditional mentor: A traditional mentor possesses extensive experience in a specific field and offers guidance, advice, and support to less experienced individuals, typically within the same profession. This form of mentorship aids professional development through tailored support and advice, making it suitable for those transitioning to new roles or seeking career advancement in their current field.
2. Peer mentor: A peer mentor operates at a career or academic level comparable to their mentees. They provide support, share insights, and offer advice based on their experiences. This mentorship emphasises collaboration and mutual growth, making it especially effective in fostering camaraderie and understanding in academic environments.
3. Reverse mentor: In reverse mentorship, a younger or less experienced person guides a senior colleague, often in technology, social media, and contemporary trends. This arrangement fosters intergenerational collaboration, introduces fresh perspectives to skilled professionals, and helps mitigate knowledge gaps in fast-changing fields, mainly when senior staff must keep abreast of new technologies and evolving workplace norms.
4. Career mentor: A career mentor focuses on aiding their mentee's professional development and career advancement, leveraging their extensive experience within a particular industry. Career mentoring assists individuals in navigating career choices, making informed decisions, and creating strategies for growth and success, making it especially useful for anyone seeking career advancement or transition at any point in their professional journey.
5. Life coach as a mentor: A life coach emphasises personal development, helping individuals define and achieve personal and professional objectives by offering guidance, motivation, and emotional support. This mentoring method provides a holistic approach to personal growth, aiding in self-discovery, confidence building, and life management skills. It is particularly suitable for those seeking clarity in life choices, individual goal setting, and overcoming challenges to succeed.

13.3.2 Mentee

A mentee is someone eager to grow, learn, and develop professionally or personally and who engages with a mentor. They are active participants in their development journey and not just mere recipients of a mentor's wisdom. The mentee's role is to be open, curious, and ready to transform the knowledge and advice they receive into meaningful progress in their career or personal life. The different types of mentees are [4]:

1. **The eager learner**: characterised by immense enthusiasm for acquiring new skills and knowledge. Often driven by the desire to excel in their current roles or broaden their expertise, they immerse themselves in learning opportunities. However, they may face challenges in focusing their efforts or applying their knowledge practically. A mentor's role for the eager learner involves providing structured learning paths, challenging their thinking, and helping them set realistic goals.
2. **The undergraduate:** They typically embark on their mentorship journey whilst navigating the complexities of university life. They often pursue academic success, career guidance, and personal growth. Balancing coursework, extracurricular activities, and early career planning, they seek mentorship that offers both academic support and insights into the professional world. A mentor for an undergraduate mentee plays a crucial role in bridging the gap between academic theories and practical applications, providing career advice, and fostering personal development. This relationship is invaluable for undergraduates shaping their future paths, often influenced by mentors guiding them through their transformative university years.
3. **The graduate:** Graduate mentees, having advanced beyond their undergraduate studies, often enter mentorship with a focus on specialised academic research or professional career development in their chosen field. They seek guidance on navigating complex research projects, academic publishing, or transitioning effectively into industry-specific roles. Mentors play a pivotal role in offering expertise in these specialised areas, providing critical feedback on research, and aiding in building professional networks. The mentor's experience is invaluable in helping graduate mentees make informed decisions about their future careers, whether in academia or the professional world.
4. **The goal-setter:** They are distinctive for their focus on specific, often ambitious, objectives. Whether aiming for career milestones, personal achievements, or academic targets, they approach mentorship with a clear vision. This type of mentee benefits greatly from a mentor who can provide strategic guidance, help in breaking down goals into manageable steps, and offer accountability. The relationship thrives on the mentor's ability to align advice and support with the mentee's defined objectives, navigating a path that is both challenging and rewarding. For the goal-setter, mentorship becomes a key tool in the journey toward achieving their set goals.

5. **The transitioner:** The transitioner mentee is typically in the midst of significant change, such as shifting careers, returning to the workforce, or transitioning to a different role within their field. They often seek mentorship to navigate the uncertainties and challenges of this change. A mentor's role is crucial in providing insights into new industries or roles, offering emotional support, and sharing strategies for adapting to change. This mentorship is invaluable in helping transitioners build confidence, acquire new skills, and successfully adapt to their new environments or roles.
6. **The explorer:** They are characterised by their curiosity and openness to diverse experiences and knowledge areas. Often unsure of their exact career path or academic focus, they seek mentorship that can provide a broad perspective and exposure to multiple possibilities. Mentors working with explorer mentees guide them through various options, help them discover their interests and strengths, and offer advice on potential paths. This mentorship is crucial in assisting explorers in finding their niche and making informed decisions about their future direction.
7. **The parent mentee:** The parent mentee often engages in mentorship whilst juggling the responsibilities of parenting with professional or personal development. They seek guidance on effectively balancing these roles, managing time, and pursuing career or educational goals amidst the unique challenges of parenthood. A mentor for a parent mentee can offer invaluable support by sharing strategies for work-life balance, providing empathetic understanding, and helping them navigate the complexities of being both a parent and a professional or student. This mentorship is crucial in empowering parent mentees to achieve their objectives without compromising their parenting commitments.
8. **The professional:** The professional mentee is typically well-established in their career but seeks mentorship for further advancement, skill enhancement, or navigating specific workplace challenges. They value mentorship that provides advanced career insights, leadership development, and strategic networking opportunities. Mentors play a key role in offering industry-specific knowledge, guidance on professional growth, and advice on managing complex workplace dynamics. This mentorship is crucial for professionals aiming to elevate their careers to the next level, whether through climbing the corporate ladder or expanding their professional capabilities.

13.4 The Mentor–Mentee Relationship

Each mentoring relationship is distinct. Yet, certain fundamental behaviours from both mentees and mentors can significantly enhance effective mentoring, regardless of the formal or informal nature of the relationship. Key behaviours include setting aligned expectations, nurturing rapport, ensuring open communication, and fostering mentee autonomy. Studies show that mentors who practice these behaviours typically have mentees who evaluate their mentoring experiences positively. Moreover, successful mentorship involves recognising diversity and prioritising equity within the relationship [2]. It flourishes when mentors and mentees cultivate trust, share each other's strengths and weaknesses, and connect personally. Some scholars describe this quality of mentorship as interpersonal comfort, which enables open dialogue and sharing of opinions without fear. Furthermore, research suggests that interpersonal dynamics and significant similarities between mentees and mentors contribute to this comfort, predicting the extent of psychosocial and career support received and offered.

13.5 The Stages of Mentoring [5]

1. **The initiation stage**: At this point, two individuals embark on a mentoring relationship. In informal mentoring, potential mentors and mentees connect through professional or social interactions. Mentees typically seek out successful, experienced individuals they admire as role models, whilst mentors look for talented individuals who are receptive to guidance. This stage in mentoring research highlights the mentee's efforts to prove their worthiness of a mentor's attention. Both parties desire a positive and enjoyable relationship that validates the commitment of time and effort in mentoring.

   In contrast, formal mentoring programmes oversee the matching process instead of allowing these relationships to form naturally. These programmes effectively take into account demographic factors and shared professional interests. The method of assigning a mentee to a mentor varies significantly between different formal mentoring programmes. In some cases, mentors review profiles and select their mentees, whilst in others, programme administrators pair mentors with mentees. Regardless of the chosen approach, a successful formal mentoring programme relies on active participation from both parties and the evaluation of the compatibility of the mentor–mentee relationship.
2. **The cultivation stage** marks the core of learning and development. Following a successful initiation stage, this phase allows the mentee to learn from the mentor. At this point, two primary mentoring functions are fully realised. The career-related function typically comes first, as the mentor guides the mentee on how to navigate their work effectively and efficiently. This coaching can occur within the mentee's organisation, where the mentor assigns challenging tasks, enhances the mentee's visibility, and actively promotes them through recognition and advancement. Mentors outside the mentee's organisation also offer valuable insights on how to succeed, despite lacking the authority to intervene directly.

   The psychosocial function develops once a strong interpersonal bond is formed between mentor and mentee. In this function, the mentor validates the mentee's professional identity, transforming the relationship into a genuine friendship.

   Overall, the cultivation stage proves beneficial for both mentor and mentee. The mentor imparts important lessons from their experiences, whilst the mentee may also teach the mentor about new technologies, methodologies, and emerging field issues.

3. **The separation stage** signifies the conclusion of a mentoring relationship and can occur for various reasons. There may be nothing more to learn, the mentee might desire to forge an independent identity, or the mentor might encourage the mentee to pursue their path, similar to how a parent would support an adult child. If both parties do not mutually acknowledge this ending, it can lead to stress, with one party struggling to cope with the change. Conflicts may arise if only one individual wishes to end the mentoring relationship. Mentees might feel abandoned, betrayed, or ill-prepared if they view the separation as too soon. Conversely, mentors might feel deceived or undervalued if the mentee no longer seeks guidance or support.
4. In the **redefinition stage**, the mentor and mentee acknowledge that their bond can persist, although it will differ from their mentoring dynamic. If they navigate the separation stage effectively, their relationship may transition into a colleague connection or a social friendship. Unlike the cultivation stage, the mentee's professional growth is no longer emphasised. The previous mentor might begin mentoring new mentees, whilst the former mentee could take on the role of a mentor to others.

13.6 Effects of Mentoring on Outcomes

A wide range of outcomes, including behavioural, attitudinal, health-related, relational, motivational, and career progression, is associated with mentoring [6].

1. **Behavioural outcomes: Mentoring leads to improvements in behaviour**
   It is widely recognised as a strategy to boost positive behaviours (like academic or job performance) and reduce negative ones (such as school dropouts or substance abuse). Formal mentoring programmes for youth and college students typically aim to support 'at-risk' individuals, hoping to prevent adverse outcomes like drug use, teen pregnancy, academic failure, and college dropouts, whilst promoting beneficial behaviours. Mentors can also influence protégé behaviour by providing practical help, such as assisting with article publications, completing homework, or successfully finishing work tasks.
2. **Attitudinal outcomes: Mentoring is linked to favourable attitudes**
   Mentoring positively influences the attitudes of protégés—as they are likely to develop favourable perceptions toward the activities they undertake with their mentors. This can encompass tasks related to graduate training or job responsibilities. Having a mentor can also strengthen their psychological attachment to their environment, be it university or workplace.
3. **Health-related outcomes: Mentoring promotes positive health impacts**
   A vital aspect of mentoring includes offering emotional and health-related support to the protégé. Mentors may provide a listening ear, offer guidance during stressful times, or counsel on personal and work-related challenges. They can boost well-being by challenging negative self-perceptions and enhancing protégés' self-confidence or self-esteem. Additionally, mentors might encourage

physical health by exercising alongside protégés or helping them access healthcare services.

4. **Relational outcomes: Mentoring nurtures positive relationship development** Mentoring can improve interactions with family and peers. Mentors may assist protégés in navigating interpersonal challenges at work or home. The close, trusting relationship with a mentor may also help protégés form constructive expectations about relationships with others, fostering positive connections.
5. **Motivational outcomes: Mentoring encourages heightened motivation** Protégé motivation and engagement can be positively affected by mentoring. Mentors expose protégés to educational and social opportunities by serving as role models, motivating them to pursue new experiences. They can also support protégés in setting practical goals and achieving personally significant outcomes whilst helping them remain focused and avoid distractions.
6. **Career outcomes: Mentoring leads to beneficial career results** Mentors share specific knowledge and skills that aid in protégé learning and development. They can also expand professional networks by connecting protégés with influential figures in academic and professional settings. These connections, including better salaries, promotions, and job offers, can be crucial for career advancement. Mentors may also expose youth and college students to various career options, facilitating exploration in this area.

13.7 Potential Problems in Mentor Relationships

Whilst mentoring is typically characterised as a beneficial relationship for both the mentee and the mentor, issues within this dynamic can impede the career growth of either party. If the boundaries of the relationship are not clearly defined, a mentee may rely excessively on the mentor, seeking micromanagement rather than guidance and support. Additionally, a mentee might request personal favours or anticipate involvement and recognition for the mentor's work. Such dynamics would hinder the mentee's independence and complicate the separation phase [7–9].

Mentors should neither manipulate nor exploit their mentees, nor should they claim ownership of the mentee's accomplishments. They might resist the separation phase, wanting a say in the mentee's career choices. Serious interpersonal problems can diminish the effectiveness of many mentoring lessons [7].

One of the most noticeable interpersonal issues arises when the relationship shifts from professional to personal. Studies on cross-gender mentoring highlight sexual relationships as a potential challenge. Suppose such personal relationships are established within a single organisation. In that case, it typically results in the termination of any formal arrangements between the two and may even lead to the dismissal of one or both individuals involved [8].

Beyond relationship-related troubles, mentors and mentees might face performance-related issues. Mentors may feel envious if their mentees excel. Furthermore, one party might be affected by mistakes made by the other. For instance, a mentee may suffer reputational damage if their mentor engages in unethical behaviour. Similarly, a mentor's reputation may suffer if their mentee fails to meet performance standards. The mentor's ability to select an appropriate mentee and the quality of their guidance may be questioned [9].

Challenges in mentoring can be alleviated when both parties have a mutual understanding of the expectations for the professional relationship. Formal mentoring programmes often incorporate training to clarify these expectations. The specific content of training programmes varies depending on the mentoring style and the objectives of the programme.

Ultimately, both parties' ongoing personal reflection on the mentor–mentee relationship—at the outset and throughout—fosters a strong, growth-focused connection. Importantly, mentors and mentees have personal aspirations and challenges in a complex environment. Everyone has difficult days, and practicing forgiveness and patience can help navigate perceived obstacles in creating a successful mentoring relationship [10].

13.8 Why Mentors in Dentistry?

Dentistry is a distinct branch of medicine as it blends a foundation in biology and dental science with specialised technical skills. Dental school is crucial for building valuable relationships and mentorships among professors, dental attenders, and students. One of the most remarkable aspects of dentistry is its continuous evolution, requiring dentists to engage in ongoing education to stay updated with the latest advancements.

Whether it is your first-year practicing dentistry or your first year after transitioning to a new practice, you will likely experience a learning curve as you adapt to the routines and protocols of your new environment. This curve can be particularly steep for those new to the field. Uncertainty about treatment planning, time management stress, and insecurity regarding technique can take a toll on your well-being. Many dentists question their career choices during the early years of practice. Practical guidance from a dedicated mentor can help you sidestep these initial challenges [11, 12].

A mentor is a seasoned practitioner committed to aiding others in enhancing their skills and growth. They provide invaluable insight gained from their own experiences. Whilst your dental school instructors worked diligently to teach you the fundamentals, certain aspects of dentistry cannot be fully grasped in a classroom. This is where a mentor steps in.

Your mentor can customise their advice based on specific situations you face. Most dental professionals, including dentists, hygienists, and assistants, struggle to balance multiple cases whilst adhering to schedules. Learning time management in a dental environment can be particularly daunting. Thankfully, a support system can help you pinpoint the right moments for switching tasks and ways to find a productive rhythm throughout your workday [13].

13.8.1 A Dentist Only Understands the Problems and Solutions

Establishing a professional connection is difficult unless you have experienced the rigours of dental school, residency, associate roles, and ownership in dentistry. Although you can share patient concerns with other professionals, only fellow dentists can genuinely grasp the stresses inherent in this field. When you find a mentor or take on that role for new dentists, you will share common ground, making it easier to navigate the unique challenges of your profession that only another dentist can appreciate [13].

13.8.2 Dentists Can Only Provide Better Feedback

Enhancing your dental skills is best achieved through constructive feedback from a dental mentor. Mentees gain insight from professionals by discussing treatment strategies, patient challenges, and successes. Exploring alternative treatment options can be tricky until you have conversed with an experienced dentist, as they have faced similar situations. Moreover, it provides a secure environment to exchange ideas or refine a proposed treatment plan [12, 13].

13.8.3 A Mentee from Dentistry Can Only Help Develop New Skills

After completing dental school and residency, acquiring new skills can pose a challenge. Participating in continuing education courses is essential for mastering new dental techniques; however, guidance from a mentor holds significant value. A general dentist can recommend paths and competencies that might be overlooked in dental school. Without an advisor, you might never consider incorporating additional advanced treatment options into your practice or enhancing your skill set. Mentees can learn techniques such as integrating recent advancements into general practice and exploring dentistry's multifaceted aspects, including education, dental research, and public health. Numerous career opportunities exist beyond clinical work that dentists can tap into, but awareness of them often requires guidance [11–13].

13.8.4 A Mentor Can Cultivate Confidence

A mentor serves as a role model to guide a new dentist in achieving their full career potential. Whether they aim to own a practice or stay as an associate, a mentor can assist their mentee by leveraging their strengths and addressing their weaknesses. The influence of mentors on dentists can be profound, offering clinical insights or practical advice for managing a successful practice. Mentoring extends beyond just practice management. It encompasses guidance on selecting beneficial continuing education courses and strategies for effectively repaying student loans [13].

13.8.5 A Mentee Can Reflect Upon a Mentor's Career

Mentoring can be empowering, allowing one dentist to teach another whilst reflecting on the highs and lows of their career. A dental mentorship is an excellent way to build both a professional and personal support network. Mentors can share their knowledge and experiences with newer dentists and encourage them to acquire valuable skills, such as orthodontics or practice management. An enthusiastic mentor can significantly impact a mentee's career by instilling self-confidence. Establishing a mentor–mentee relationship opens the door to invaluable lessons, making it fulfilling to learn from a colleague. Ultimately, you will discover your full potential as a dentist, and this experience will serve as a guide, helping you foster a meaningful career [11–13].

13.9 Dental Mentorship: How This Work?

Dental mentors should be open to sharing insights from their professional experiences. They ought to elaborate on their unique approaches to business, practice management, and patient care, which can help the mentee in developing their style. Whilst each mentor varies, mentors can assist in various ways, including [13]:

- Evaluating your cases
- Providing constructive feedback
- Clarifying professional ethics
- Addressing workplace challenges
- Suggesting methods to enhance specific skills, or
- Recommending strategies to reach your professional objectives

Mentorship can be an invaluable support system for a mentee during their first, often daunting, year as a dental practitioner. Finding time to discuss operational methods and best practices with colleagues can be challenging in a busy practice. A mentor can act as both a guide and a sounding board, especially for novices who may feel uncertain or pressured to excel. Additionally, engaging with your mentor can help alleviate the isolation in your daily practice.

13.10 Finding the Right Mentor

Finding a trustworthy mentor who is experienced, whose insights resonate with you, or who specialises in a field that sparks your interest is essential. Your mentor could be a senior colleague at your workplace, a professor or supervisor from your university, someone whose work you respect and follow, a recommendation from a peer, or a connection established through a mentorship programme offered by professional organisations. A mentorship often begins with a conversation [14]. To identify the right mentor [15]:

- Connect with individuals in your areas of interest or specific practices.
- Initiate a conversation—inquire about their experiences and approaches. You will quickly sense whether a mentor–mentee relationship could develop between you.
- Ask for recommendations—seek introductions from friends and colleagues, as these can be more effective and less daunting than cold outreach.
- Consult your professional association for guidance.

13.11 Getting More Out of Mentorship

Mentorship differs from a lecture, as it requires you to engage actively rather than just passively absorbing information. Bring your ideas, questions, and work experiences into the mix to maximise the arrangement [16]. You could:

- Shadow your mentor and observe their effective practices.
- Outline your goals for the mentorship, current job, and future career.
- Pose detailed inquiries about procedures, protocols, or problem-solving strategies.
- Seek insights on the best approaches, potential pitfalls, and key considerations.
- Request candid feedback.
- Inquire about what you can offer in return—are there skills or knowledge you can share with your mentor?
- Show appreciation; let your mentor know how crucial they have been to your professional journey.
- Respectfully agree to disagree sometimes, honouring the mentor–mentee relationship you have fostered.

13.12 Essentials of Successful Mentorship

13.12.1 Knowledge

Trust, openness, and constructive support are vital qualities in every mentor, which can only be achieved if the mentor possesses a sufficient understanding of themselves. This self-awareness is crucial for managing their behaviours when assisting others. Conducting a personal SWOT (strengths, weaknesses, opportunities, and threats) analysis can be valuable for identifying one's strengths and weaknesses. A mentor should align with the mentee's objectives to remain effective, necessitating behavioural awareness and emotional intelligence to understand others [4].

Providing emotional guidance requires an empathetic approach, demonstrating care and respect for the mentee. As a mentor, it is essential to approach the relationship with empathy to offer emotional guidance toward the mentee's goals. This guidance is informed by the mentee's feelings (affective) and the experiences (cognitive) that shape those feelings. Empathetic mentors are more capable of fostering the intimacy and trust that are critical to the psychosocial aspects of mentoring [17]. Snowden et al. expand on Darwin's dimensions of the mentoring personality, emphasising the key behaviours dental care professionals identify that as contributing to a successful mentoring relationship [18]. These behaviours, listed in descending order of significance, include approachability, communication, non-bias, patience, enthusiasm, trust, empathy, motivation, willingness, reflection, negotiation, friendliness, empowerment, and leadership. These features suggest that mentees have a preference for nurturing mentors, which is unsurprising considering the profession of dentists routinely cares for its patients.

13.12.2 Communication

Effective interpersonal communication fosters successful mentoring and includes verbal and non-verbal aspects. Non-verbal communication encompasses facial expressions, gestures, posture, body orientation, and spatial use. It's believed that non-verbal cues often communicate deeper meaning than words alone, and a mentor's ability to interpret these subtle signals from mentees is crucial, as they indicate the level of engagement [19]. Egan suggested positioning yourself 'squarely' facing the mentee, utilising an 'open' posture, 'leaning' in towards them, maintaining 'eye' contact, and remaining 'relaxed' (acronym SOLER) to increase engagement [20].

Active listening is essential for grasping the mentee's intentions and emotions whilst uncovering the actual message they wish to communicate. A mentor must set aside judgment, remain open-minded, and accept the mentee's words without rushing to offer solutions or take control. A mentor must interpret both the spoken and underlying meanings to achieve deeper insight and comprehension. In addition to listening, posing thoughtful and open-ended questions fosters rapport, grants mentees the freedom to express themselves, and encourages open dialogue [21]. Hypothetical questions can present scenarios that facilitate the exploration of new ideas or concepts without leading to confrontation, thus avoiding defensiveness. Probing questions can extract additional information, clarify existing thought processes, or be helpful when mentees are reluctant to share. Socratic questioning promotes reflection on actions and feelings, seeks clarification, affirms active listening, encourages mentee elaboration, and reassures them that their thoughts are valued. However, it is crucial to use questioning judiciously, ensuring that the mentee possesses the necessary skills and understanding to respond appropriately [21].

13.12.3 Responsibilities

The European Mentoring and Coaching Council (EMCC) Code of Ethics establishes standards for mentors, ensuring accountability, best practices, and professional competence in their work. It encompasses competence, context, boundary management, integrity, and professionalism [22]. The International Coaching Federation (ICF) Code of Ethics emphasises the mentor's obligation to the mentee, particularly in fostering a beneficial relationship under the banner of 'responsibility to the client'. Before their first meeting, mentors must help mentees understand the nature and significance of their relationship. The ICF views mentoring as a collaborative partnership where both parties clearly understand their roles and responsibilities. Hence, mentors should strive to build an alliance with the mentee that guarantees high-quality mentoring, free from biases related to race, gender, or other differences [23].

Mentors must uphold trust and confidentiality to foster an open and safe environment. This extends to all meeting notes, whether written or electronic and to how information is shared among all participants. It is crucial to address the boundaries of confidentiality right from the beginning and include them in the contract, along with any potential conflicts of interest.

13.13 Best Practices for Successful Mentoring

1. **Effective planning and preparation** necessitate dedicating time to establishing clear objectives, timelines, and methods that align with organisational goals and participants' needs. Ambiguous goals and objectives can cause confusion and lack of direction, making it difficult for mentors and mentees to comprehend their roles and expectations. Without clear guidance, participants may find it challenging to engage effectively, thereby reducing the programme's potential for significant growth and development [24].
2. **Thoughtful pairing of mentors and mentees**: A successful programme considers the compatibility of mentor–mentee pairs, evaluating factors such as skills, experience, personality, and goals to foster productive relationships. Neglecting the critical aspect of properly matching mentors and mentees can lead to mismatched expectations, differing communication styles, or unmet developmental needs [24].
3. **Emphasis on diversity, equity, inclusion, and belonging (DEIB):** Successful programmes acknowledge the value of diverse perspectives and experiences, actively creating inclusive environments where all participants feel appreciated and supported. Ignoring DEIB considerations risks perpetuating biases, excluding underrepresented groups, and creating barriers to participation and engagement [24].
4. **Leadership endorsement and support**: Effective mentoring programmes gain backing from organisational leaders who provide resources, visibility, and

endorsement, which reinforces the programme's credibility and cultivates a culture of learning and development [24].

5. **Monitoring progress and assessing outcomes:** Effective programmes implement systems to track the progress of mentor–mentee relationships, gather feedback, and evaluate the impact of mentoring on participant development and organisational objectives, facilitating ongoing improvement and accountability. Failing to create mechanisms for monitoring progress and assessing outcomes makes it challenging to evaluate the programme's effectiveness, identify improvement areas, and justify ongoing investment [24].

13.14 Current Perspectives

The definition of mentoring has been expanded to go beyond a relationship between two individuals—a dyadic mentoring relationship—to include a broad array of additional constructs and relationships [2]. This expansion has come about through the recognition that, in many cases, there are more efficient and more effective ways for mentees to develop wisdom and expertise than by having it imparted by a single mentor and that one mentor is not likely to fulfil all of a mentee's needs. Moving beyond the 'one mentor–one mentee' approach to mentoring relationships becomes especially critical in contexts where relatively few mentors are available to meet the mentoring requirements of many mentees or when one mentor cannot meet all the mentoring commitments of a particular mentee [2].

13.15 Conclusions

Mentors possess extensive experience and knowledge, providing a range of organisational and interpersonal skills that benefit both individuals and organisations. They improve mentees' self-awareness and represent a cost-effective investment in personal and professional development, ultimately enhancing patient care safety. Our primary mission is to ensure safer patient care beyond simple compliance with checklists. By integrating evidence-based dentistry into our clinical practice, we must acknowledge the recognised benefits from the corporate sector: effective mentorship. Nonetheless, it's essential to understand that a mentor can only facilitate transformational change when paired with a willing mentee. Just like mentees, mentors also require training and development, which is made possible only if the employing organisation values mentorship and promotes a culture that nurtures the essential qualities of those looking to mentor others.

References

1. https://dictionary.cambridge.org/dictionary/english/mentor - Accessed 25 Mar 2025
2. National Academies of Sciences, Engineering, and Medicine, Policy and Global Affairs, Board on Higher Education and Workforce, Committee on Effective Mentoring in STEMM. In: Dahlberg ML, Byars-Winston A, editors. The science of effective mentorship in STEMM. Washington, DC: National Academies Press (US); 2019. The Science of Mentoring Relationships: What Is Mentorship? Available from: https://www.ncbi.nlm.nih.gov/books/NBK552775/.
3. https://ideas.ted.com/the-5-types-of-mentors-you-need-in-your-life/. Accessed 25 Mar 2025
4. https://www.togetherplatform.com/blog/mentor-vs-mentee. Accessed 25 Mar 2025
5. Chao GT. Mentoring phases and outcomes. J Vocat Behav. 1997;51(1):15–28.
6. Eby LT, Allen TD, Evans SC, Ng T, Dubois D. Does mentoring matter? A multidisciplinary meta-analysis comparing mentored and non-mentored individuals. J Vocat Behav. 2008;72(2):254–67. https://doi.org/10.1016/j.jvb.2007.04.005. PMID: 19343074; PMCID: PMC2352144
7. https://mentorloop.com/blog/6-common-mentoring-challenges-solutions/. Accessed 25 Mar 2025
8. https://www.womentech.net/blog/6-common-challenges-in-mentoring-relationships#:~:text=6%20Common%20Challenges%20in%20Mentoring%20Relationships%20*,from%20Others:%20*%20Mismatch%20of%20Mentoring%20Pairs: Accessed 25 Mar 2025
9. https://scse.d.umn.edu/addressing-challenges. Accessed 25 Mar 2025
10. https://www.apa.org/education-career/grad/mentoring. Accessed 25 Mar 2025
11. https://www.communitydentalpartners.com/articles/mentorship-in-dentistry/. Accessed 25 Mar 2025
12. https://dentistry.co.uk/2024/02/23/the-power-of-mentoring-in-dentistry/. Accessed 25 Mar 2025
13. https://orthodontics.com/importance-of-a-mentor-in-the-dental-world/. Accessed 25 Mar 2025
14. https://www.interfolio.com/resources/blog/five-insights-when-selecting-a-mentor/. Accessed 25 Mar 2025
15. https://www.indeed.com/career-advice/career-development/why-is-a-mentor-important. Accessed 25 Mar 2025
16. https://www.togetherplatform.com/blog/examples-of-mentoring-program-goals. Accessed 25 Mar 2025
17. Leck J, Orser B. Fostering trust in mentoring relationships: an exploratory study. Equal Divers Inclusion Int J. 2013;32(4):410–25.
18. Snowden M, Ellwood F, McSherry R, Halsall J, Hough D. Mentoring and you. Dent Nurs. 2016;12(7):386–91.
19. Papadopoulos R. The role of non verbal communication in effective teaching and learning. Doctoral dissertation, University of Oxford.
20. Egan G. The skilled helper: a systematic approach to effective helping. 4th ed. Brooks-Cole; 1990.
21. Zachary LJ. The mentor's guide: facilitating effective learning relationships. Wiley; 2011.
22. Passmore J, Brown H, Csigas Z. The state of play in European coaching & mentoring. Henley Business School; 2017.
23. van der Hoorn S, Perfetto C, Bekker C. Mentor coaching. InSolution focused coaching supervision. Routledge; 2024. p. 144–58.
24. https://chronus.com/how-to-start-a-mentoring-program. Accessed 25 Mar 2025

Workplace-Based Assessment and Feedback in Dental Sciences Education

14

R. Sajith Kumar

14.1 Introduction

Education in general and health sciences education particularly is undergoing paradigm shifts at present. The pattern of education is now getting adapted to student-friendly initiatives which also incorporate closeness to real-life environments. Competency Based or outcome based education is the norm of the day. The students of dental sciences are expected to perform various tasks through structurally acquired skills. However due to various reasons, the training for these skills and sometimes assessment takes place in artificial settings. The importance of simulation in skills training need not be overemphasised.

Assessment of learning and skills acquisition is conventionally carried out at specific times and environments. These are usually fragmented and detached from the scenarios the graduate should expect in real life. Unusual cases and topics are selected for examinations. Students are usually under pressure due to obvious reasons. The environments and personnel involved are less likely to be friendly, if not frightening. The thought of consequences of incomplete performances are often threatening for the minds of students and hinder their performances. Lack of variety of day-to-day encounters, fewer unfamiliar examiners and limited time are major weaknesses in the conventional assessment system which also happens to be mostly summative [1].

The *Miller's Pyramid* of acquiring competence and Miller's Framework on clinical assessment are based on professional practice requirements rather than on artificial academic or testing environments [2]. The ascendance from purely cognitive levels like 'Knows and Knows How' to behavioural levels like 'Shows and Shows How' is well explained therein. The graduate is expected to reach the performance

R. Sajith Kumar (✉)
Department of Infectious Diseases, Convener NMC Nodal Centre for Faculty Development, Government Medical College, Kottayam, Kerala, India

Academic Staff College, Kerala University of Health Sciences, Thrissur, Kerala, India

R. M. Baiju, S. Thomas (eds.), *The Dental Teacher*,
https://doi.org/10.1007/978-3-032-07551-2_14

level (Does) when he is out of the campus and serving the community. Even though the students and interns demonstrate various skills and tasks whilst inside the campus, they are almost always under the supervision of the teachers and hence qualify to be under the 'Shows How' region only. Competency can be understood as the habitual and judicious use of communication, knowledge, technical skills, clinical reasoning, emotions, values, and reflection in daily practice for the benefit of the individual and community being served [2].

Workplace-based assessment aims to engage the students whilst they are practising the skills [3]. This modality is an integral part of competency assessment; the student is watched at his comfort and convenience without specific examination settings. This gives ample opportunities for the teacher as well as the student to get going without significant changes in work or study schedules. This form of assessment is expected to take place on a day-to-day basis but with specific objectives. This is mostly used for formative assessment taking place during the training phase itself. The student's strengths and weaknesses are identified, leading to greater insights for both students and teachers regarding specific performance gaps on both sides. These performance gaps are identified as the gap between the quality of expected and actual acts. Recognition of these gaps whilst at work and adequate responses aimed at minimising the gaps is the major concept behind WPBA [3].

Whilst the teacher and student are attending daily activities, they are observed and assessed. The assessment has to be reliable and valid. Observation of the student's performance is the key attribute of WPBA. This observation may be done by a regular teacher in usual teaching-learning environments like mini-clinical examination in an outpatient clinic or ward. It may be based on assessment of students over a period of time, including past activities like filed case sheets, OP charts, etc. It can also be direct or indirect observation by many stakeholders including feedback from patients, staff nurses etc. The last type based on feedback from various sources (multi-source feedback) is referred to as 360-degree assessment and is perhaps the best of all.

There are many WPBA tools used across the world; the most commonly used tools in WPBA can be divided into four categories:

1. Observation of clinical activities—mini-CEX and DOPS
2. Discussion of clinical cases—such as CSR and the CBD
3. Documentation of work experience through logbooks—such as clinical encounter cards
4. Feedback from peers, coworkers, and patients—MSF/360° mini-PAT, team assessment of behaviours, and the patient satisfaction questionnaire

Mini-clinical Evaluation Exercise (mini-CEx) This is the most commonly used and easier method. This was originally introduced by Norcini in 1995 in the United States for formative assessment of medical students and interns and has become a regular practice in many countries [4]. During the regular work in a dental clinic or ward rounds, the student examines a real patient in front of a teacher. The assessment in areas of history taking, physical examination, clinical judgement, communication skills, professionalism, documentation etc., can be included one at a time or in combination. The teacher observes the performance (behaviour) of the student (usually one at a time) and provides immediate feedback. A standardised checklist is used to mark the observations and to note the suggestions. The student also does a self-appraisal and this can be compared with that of the teacher. The gaps and good things are shared immediately and the document filed. The student is always given a chance to make remediation and improve his performance on a later date, when the scene gets repeated. The sessions take place during regular activity, but at a time convenient and comfortable for both teacher and student. The reliability increases with more and more sessions. Usually 4–14 sessions are conducted each lasting for 5–15 min [4]. The improvement over a period can be documented and can form part of the logbook entries as well. The cases can be chosen based on the variety that is available and the students will have the option to hold the sessions with different teachers also. Of course, the teachers also need training and must take care to be non-judgmental as well as non-threatening.

Clinical Encounter Cards Initiated in McMaster University in Canada, CEC lets the students to be assessed periodically based on the student's performance in various dimensions like case taking including history, physical examination, professionalism, behaviour, skill, case presentation, diagnosis and treatment [3]. The small size cards will document the level of student's actions as unsatisfactory, below or above expectations outstanding, professional etc. The teacher will also record the feedback at the end of the session. Hatala and Norman have documented that it is a feasible, valid and reliable method if eight or more encounters are documented. Each session may last up to 20 min including feedback.

Direct Observation of Procedural Skills (DOPSs) Dental students are expected to perform many tasks based on the skills training that they receive from the first year onwards in skill labs and by observing their teachers through methods like DOAP (Demonstrate, Observe, Assist, Perform). In DOPS a procedure involved in patient care is performed by the student under the observation of the teacher in the usual clinical setting [5]. Various parameters involved in patient care like attitudes, communication and psychomotor domains like manual dexterity, proper handling of instruments, infection control practices etc. are addressed. Usually a checklist resembling the OSCE (Objective Structured Clinical Examination) depicting the steps in a procedure is used to assess and confirm that the student is following all steps in a structured and systematic manner. DOPS is usually conducted after the students have demonstrated their ability in a mannequin or model and have gone through sufficient clinical trainings. Competency Based Dental Education or Competency Based Dynamic Curriculum in India expects the students to be able to demonstrate EPAs (Entrustable Professional Achievements). DOPS is one of the prerequisites needed to be completed before the student achieves the competency needed to perform EPAs [6]. The DOPS scoring is usually given as having achieved the competency or not. The assessor variability is a factor influencing DOPS assessment. More the number of DOPS sessions for each skill, the closer the student will be to achieving competency. DOPS is also useful as a summative assessment tool, when performed in routine clinical settings. Achieving competency is not proved by demonstration in one skill or competency alone and must be completed in as many situations as possible. Performance at one time also may not be replicable and therefore repeated sessions are recommended for each skill.

Blinded Patient Encounters This is similar to a short case discussion, where the student is allotted a patient, whose details are not shared and hence the term 'blinded'. This can be conducted with a group of students also, where one student will take the lead and discuss the case. Attributes of history taking, examination, management plans, treatment options etc. can be included. The details of the case are unblinded by the teacher at the end and the students are given scores.

Case-Based Discussion In this form of WPBA, the patient is worked up by the student under the supervision of the teacher and then discussed when attributes like clinical judgement, decision making, treatment planning etc. can be assessed. This is also called as CSR (Case Sheet Review). The relevant investigations, radiographs etc. will form part of discussion [3]. The session will be akin to a ward rounds scenario but on a one to one basis. Feedback can help the student plan the case management in future. The student may work up many cases and the teacher can select them one by one as well.

Multi-source Feedback This is also referred to as 360 degree assessment. In this activity, student's or intern's routine activities are observed directly or indirectly by many stakeholders including teacher, patient, nurses and even peers. The input from all of them are utilised to ensure that the student is made aware of the shortfalls that happen during routine work and to assist in improving the professional practices over a period of time. This is not restricted to specific patient encounters and therefore the stress experienced by the student is reduced. Standardised feedback questionnaires are used. The assessors should undergo systematic briefing before they start assessing and inter personal or interdisciplinary conflicts must be avoided. Interprofessional education is happening in many campuses and the services of various categories of personnel can be used for MSF. Mini-PAT (Mini Peer Assessment Tool) is a format for performing MSF in health care scenarios in which senior consultants; junior faculty, nurses and paramedics are involved in assessment [1]. The student can also judge his performance during the said period and collate with that of others. Quality of clinical care, accuracy of clinical practice, quality of teaching and training, facilitation of relationships with patients, relatives, colleagues etc. are usually covered [6]. An overall assessment can also be included. Anonymity is insisted and the assigned trainer discusses the feedback with student. At the end of each session, discussions are needed and preferably followed by the development of an action plan with responsibilities shared by the teacher and student. The session needs to be repeated at least twice a year.

The workplace-based assessments are not a substitute to the existing assessment methods but can act as complementary in formative assessment. Since many components are still not standardised, the validity and outcome can be questionable. The senior teachers and clinical situations will add value and reliability to these processes, as subjectivity is a major quality ascribed to these. However, their value is high as a concurrent tool which is to be used effectively by trained personnel. The occasional chance of a good student becoming over confident and a less learned student getting dejected exists.

Feedback Health Sciences Education needs lot of inputs from teachers who are experienced in training and assessment of students. Even though subjectivity is not a good quality of assessment, feedback from senior teachers, junior faculty and peers do play a major role in the development of a professional health care worker [7]. Achievement of competency and entrustment must be ensured in all graduates. Ideally it should be a two way description of a student's performance intended to guide future performance. Feedback is not a casual process but a systematised intervention plan aimed not only about the previous performance but also including action plans aimed at improvement. Without feedback, mistakes go uncorrected, good performance is not reinforced, and clinical competence is achieved empirically or, not at all. Feedback should discuss 'What was done well', 'what could be done better' and 'what could be done' to improve next time.

Feedback can be explained as the transmission of specific information about the comparison between a trainees' observed performance and a standard, given with the intent to improve the trainee's performance. Feedback therefore requires a standard which can be defined very differently as a horizon of expectation; through the performance of a reference group of colleagues or learners; through the previous performance of the learners themselves or through the opinion of the teachers about what the learners should be able to do. The criteria can be objective or subjective, absolute or relative.

Feedback must happen in many ways. It can be oral or written and can be regular or incident-based. It can be formal or informal. Formal feedback must be a regular component of all workplace-based assessments. It should be (i) specific, (ii) immediate, (iii) non-judgemental, (iv) based on first-hand information, and (v) regulated and direct [7]. It should focus on changeable behaviour and must suggest changes that can be implemented. It should not be too broad and generalised. Feedback should ideally be delivered individually and periodically. Group feedback is not recommended. Feedback should be directed towards the behaviour and not the individual. Reflections by the student and teacher at the end of the feedback will encourage constructive feedback in subsequent sessions. Feedback can be brief following every clinical contact, formative following an event or major usually done halfway through a learning process aimed at mid-course corrections. The feedback process can concentrate on promotion of the good and prevention of the worse. It is noticed that negative feedback increases motivation and performance (prevention focus group) but also that positive feedback may have a negative impact on both motivation and performance (promotion group).

The feedback can involve [7]:

(a) Task-learning processes covering the processes that are necessary to complete a task
(b) Task-motivation processes covering effort management to ensure that effort is increased until the discrepancy with standards is eliminated
(c) Meta-task processes which facilitate self-regulation and self-improvement

Sandwich method is one in which the feedback starts with appreciation, unpleasant comments, followed by unpleasant comments and encouragement. A modified version is Ask-Tell-Ask method, where the student is probed to identify his status, followed by the teacher's assessment and finally getting a commitment from the student. ADAPT model is an acronym for Ask-Discuss-Ask-Plan Together which is self-explanatory. The R2C2 model covers the importance of relationships, reactions, content and coaching in feedback. The Educational Alliance Model speaks about trusting teacher-trainee relationships, safe learning environment, regular direct observation and shared understanding between teachers and learners about the process and content of feedback and suggests a feedback culture to be developed in institutions.

A common model for giving feedback was developed by Pendleton (1998). The steps are:

- Check the learner wants feedback and he/she is ready for feedback
- Let the learner give comments/background to the material that is being assessed
- The learner states what was done well
- The observer says what was done well
- The learner says what could have been done well
- The observer states how it could be improved
- An action plan for improvement is made

The following are variables that influence better feedback:

- Use of rubrics increases the reliability of scoring and facilitates feedback communication
- Similarities in the cultural backgrounds of the provider and recipient
- The receiver's self-esteem
- Low initial skill
- Goal-setting behaviour of the learner
- Feedback as part of a multifaceted intervention (audits, outreach)

- Frequent feedback
- Rating tasks of lower complexity

In general, feedback should be:

Specific	not	General
Immediate	not	Delayed
Behavioral	not	Inferential
Descriptive	not	Evaluative
Asked for	not	Pushed Upon

References

1. Manekar V. Workplace based assessment (WPBA) in dental education- a review. J Educ Technol Health Sci. 2018; https://doi.org/10.18231/2393-8005.2018.0016.
2. Miller GE. The assessment of clinical skills /competence /performance. Acad Med. 1990:s63–7.
3. Singh T, Sood R. Workplace-based assessment: Measuring and shaping clinical learning. Natl Med J India. 2013;26:42–6.
4. Norcini JJ, Blank LL, Duffy FD, Fortna GS. The mini CEX: a method for assessing clinical skills. Ann Int Med. 2003;138:476–81.
5. Grieveson B, Kirton JA, Palmer N, Balmer MC. Evaluation of workplace based assessment tools in dental foundation training. Br Dent J. 2011;211:E8.
6. Hatala R, Norman GR. In-training evaluation during an Internal Medicine clerkship. Acad Med. 1999;74:S118–20.
7. Van de Ridder JM, Stokking KM, McGaghie WC, ten Gate OT. What is feedback in clinical education? Med Educ. 2008;42(2):189–97. https://doi.org/10.1111/j.1365-2923.2007.02973.

MIX
Papier aus verantwortungsvollen Quellen
Paper from responsible sources
FSC® C105338

If you have any concerns about our products,
you can contact us on
ProductSafety@springernature.com

In case Publisher is established outside the EU,
the EU authorized representative is:
Springer Nature Customer Service Center GmbH
Europaplatz 3, 69115 Heidelberg, Germany

Printed by Libri Plureos GmbH
in Hamburg, Germany